The AIDS Crisis

ISSUES

Volume 164

Series Editor

Lisa Firth

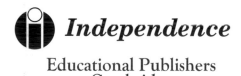

Independence

Educational Publishers
Cambridge

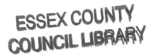
First published by Independence
The Studio, High Green
Great Shelford
Cambridge CB22 5EG
England

© Independence 2009

British Library Cataloguing in Publication Data

The AIDS Crisis – (Issues Series)
I. AIDS (Disease) II. Firth, Lisa
616.9'792

ISBN 978 1 86168 468 4

Printed in Great Britain

MWL Print Group Ltd

Cover

The illustration on the front cover is by
Simon Kneebone.

CONTENTS

Chapter One: The AIDS Epidemic

Chapter Two: HIV/AIDS in the UK

Chapter Three: Fighting HIV and AIDS

Useful information for readers

Dear Reader,

Issues: The AIDS Crisis

AIDS, the disease caused by the HIV virus, has been described as a pandemic, causing around 3 million deaths worldwide every year. Positive HIV diagnoses are also rising in the UK. What causes HIV and how can we protect ourselves against it? How do those living with the illness cope with issues such as medical treatment, stigma and discrimination? What can be done to combat AIDS in the developing world? These are some of the questions posed by **The AIDS Crisis**.

The purpose of Issues

The AIDS Crisis is the one hundred and sixty-fourth volume in the **Issues** series. The aim of this series is to offer up-to-date information about important issues in our world. Whether you are a regular reader or new to the series, we do hope you find this book a useful overview of the many and complex issues involved in the topic.

Titles in the **Issues** series are resource books designed to be of especial use to those undertaking project work or requiring an overview of facts, opinions and information on a particular subject, particularly as a prelude to undertaking their own research.

The information in this book is not from a single author, publication or organisation; the value of this unique series lies in the fact that it presents information from a wide variety of sources, including:

⇨ Government reports and statistics
⇨ Newspaper articles and features
⇨ Information from think-tanks and policy institutes
⇨ Magazine features and surveys
⇨ Website material
⇨ Literature from lobby groups and charitable organisations.*

Critical evaluation

Because the information reprinted here is from a number of different sources, readers should bear in mind the origin of the text and whether the source is likely to have a particular bias or agenda when presenting information (just as they would if undertaking their own research). It is hoped that, as you read about the many aspects of the issues explored in this book, you will critically evaluate the information presented. It is important that you decide whether you are being presented with facts or opinions. Does the writer give a biased or an unbiased report? If an opinion is being expressed, do you agree with the writer?

The AIDS Crisis offers a useful starting point for those who need convenient access to information about the many issues involved. However, it is only a starting point. Following each article is a URL to the relevant organisation's website, which you may wish to visit for further information.

Kind regards,

Lisa Firth
Editor, **Issues** series

*Please note that Independence Publishers has no political affiliations or opinions on the topics covered in the **Issues** series, and any views quoted in this book are not necessarily those of the publisher or its staff.*

HIV/AIDS

Information from Bupa

Human Immunodeficiency Virus (HIV) is an infection. It's passed from person to person via unprotected sex, from needles contaminated with infected blood, through blood transfusion or organ donation from people with the virus, and from mother to baby.

AIDS (Acquired Immune Deficiency Syndrome) is diagnosed when the immune system has been weakened so much by HIV that it can't fight certain life-threatening infections and illnesses.

Worldwide figures estimate that over 40 million people are living with HIV and around three million people die each year from AIDS-related illnesses.

HIV in the UK

The number of people living with HIV in the UK has increased steadily since the 1980s when the virus was discovered. Official figures for 2005 put this at nearly 63,500 people.

Most HIV infections in the UK occur in homosexual men. Transmission of the virus through heterosexual contact has significantly increased in recent years. However, the majority of these infections are in people who have come to live in

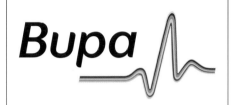

the UK from countries where HIV is widespread and have been diagnosed since living in the UK.

HIV and the immune system

The immune system protects your body against infection. A key part is white blood cells. These cells find and destroy invading germs, such as bacteria and viruses, preventing the development of serious diseases and damage to your body. HIV avoids being destroyed by the immune system by repeatedly changing its outer 'coat'. It multiplies (replicates) within the special type of white blood cells called CD4 cells. These cells are normally involved in helping other types of immune cell to attack and destroy disease-causing germs.

As HIV multiplies, it destroys CD4 cells, so there are less of them. The reduction in CD4 cells means that the body's ability to fight infection is weakened.

Causes

HIV can only be passed to someone else when the levels of the virus are high enough in the blood or other body fluids and are passed to another person.

HIV infection can be passed via blood, semen, breast milk and vaginal fluids. Therefore, you can pass or have HIV passed to you during unprotected anal or vaginal sex.

There is a small chance of infection through unprotected oral sex. It's estimated around three in every 100 homosexual men with HIV get it through unprotected oral sex with a man who has HIV. The risk of oral transmission from women is extremely low.

The virus can be passed from mother to baby if she has HIV during pregnancy, childbirth or when breastfeeding. HIV can also be passed on if you use infected needles for injections, piercings or tattoos.

HIV is not found in high enough levels in other body fluids such as saliva, sweat, urine or on the skin to cause an infection from contact with these fluids.

HIV can't be passed on through normal day-to-day activities, such as sharing cutlery, sitting on toilet seats or by shaking hands.

HIV and blood or organ donation
In the past, people have become infected with HIV through blood or organ donations. All donations in the UK are now screened for HIV, so the chances of this happening are extremely low.

Symptoms

The period immediately after a person becomes infected with HIV is called primary HIV infection. At this point you are very infectious because the level of the virus will be high in the blood. You will have symptoms of

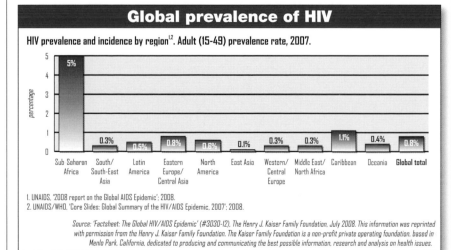

Global prevalence of HIV

HIV prevalence and incidence by region[1,2]. Adult (15-49) prevalence rate, 2007.

Sub Saharan Africa	5%
South/South-East Asia	0.3%
Latin America	0.5%
Eastern Europe/Central Asia	0.8%
North America	0.6%
East Asia	0.1%
Western/Central Europe	0.3%
Middle East/North Africa	0.3%
Caribbean	1.1%
Oceania	0.4%
Global total	0.8%

1. UNAIDS, '2008 report on the Global AIDS Epidemic', 2008.
2. UNAIDS/WHO, 'Core Slides: Global Summary of the HIV/AIDS Epidemic, 2007', 2008.

Source: 'Factsheet: The Global HIV/AIDS Epidemic' (#3030-12), The Henry J. Kaiser Family Foundation, July 2008. This information was reprinted with permission from the Henry J. Kaiser Family Foundation. The Kaiser Family Foundation is a non-profit private operating foundation, based in Menlo Park, California, dedicated to producing and communicating the best possible information, research and analysis on health issues.

HIV infection but you may miss them because they are like other infections such as flu. Early symptoms usually start about two to six weeks after the infection and last approximately five to 10 days. Some symptoms may last longer.

Signs of primary HIV include:
⇨ fever
⇨ swollen glands
⇨ sore throat
⇨ rash on the body or face
⇨ painful muscles or joints
⇨ headache
⇨ feeling sick and vomiting
⇨ ulcers on the mouth, genitals and oesophagus (tube that goes to the stomach).

More serious symptoms include heavy bleeding if you are injured. Rarely, brain infections such as meningitis can affect people with HIV infection.

Worldwide figures estimate that over 40 million people are living with HIV and around three million people die each year from AIDS-related illnesses

---

After the early symptoms, HIV may remain undetected for a number of years until your body's ability to fight infections is reduced. When this happens the number of cells which fight infections has decreased so much that your immune system can't function properly. This leaves the body vulnerable to infections. If a person develops certain life-threatening illnesses it is known as AIDS or advanced HIV disease.

AIDS
Once the immune system has been damaged, infections appear. Common infections include a type of pneumonia called pneumocystis, and tuberculosis.

Other AIDS-related illnesses can include:
⇨ various cancers
⇨ fungal, bacterial or viral in-fections

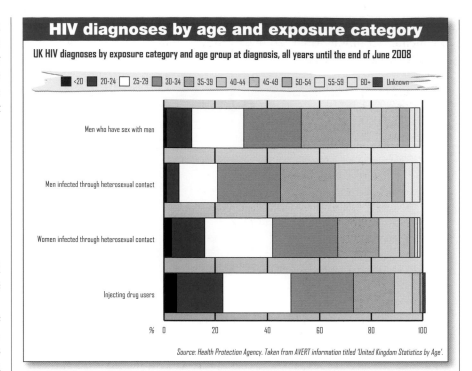

HIV diagnoses by age and exposure category

UK HIV diagnoses by exposure category and age group at diagnosis, all years until the end of June 2008

Legend: <20 | 20-24 | 25-29 | 30-34 | 35-39 | 40-44 | 45-49 | 50-54 | 55-59 | 60+ | Unknown

Categories (bars): Men who have sex with men; Men infected through heterosexual contact; Women infected through heterosexual contact; Injecting drug users

% 0 20 40 60 80 100

Source: Health Protection Agency. Taken from AVERT information titled 'United Kingdom Statistics by Age'.

⇨ sight problems
⇨ dementia.

Diagnosis
It's important to have an HIV test if you think you have been at risk of HIV infection. There are powerful and effective treatments that slow the virus. Early diagnosis can help ensure you get the best treatment so you can live a full and active life.

To test for HIV, blood is taken. HIV testing in the laboratory involves looking at a blood sample for HIV antibodies, the body's defence chemicals produced in response to infection. Testing can be done four to six weeks after infection but the virus may not be detected in the blood for up to three months in some people.

Testing is usually carried out at genitourinary medicine (GUM) clinics, where sexually transmitted infections are diagnosed and treated. Sometimes results are available after a week, some clinics offer same-day HIV testing.

Before you have a blood test for HIV you may be able to see a counsellor. The test can be explained and the implications of a possible positive diagnosis discussed. You can also talk about the test results with your GP or a counsellor.

Treatment
There is no cure for HIV infection, but treatment with anti-HIV medicines

dramatically slows the progress of the disease and has significantly reduced the number of deaths caused by AIDS-related illnesses. When used appropriately and taken properly, anti-HIV medicines can mean a person with HIV has a near-normal life expectancy.

HIV treatment is managed by specialist outpatient clinics, staffed by doctors, nurses and other health professionals. The status of your immune system and your general health is reviewed on a regular basis.

Usually, once the number of CD4 white blood cells has fallen to a low level, or if the amount of virus in your blood is very high, your specialist will recommend starting drug treatment. Treatment may be started if you develop a serious infection.

Medication
Current treatments prevent the virus from replicating in the body. This in turn reduces the amount of virus in the blood and allows the immune system to recover. To achieve this, three antiretroviral medicines are usually taken together. They normally have to be taken once a day but some need to be taken up to three times a day and at specific times. This combination therapy is termed highly active antiretroviral therapy (HAART) and has dramatically cut the number of deaths from AIDS-related illnesses since its introduction. There are

HIV/AIDS

Information from Bupa

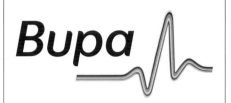

Human Immunodeficiency Virus (HIV) is an infection. It's passed from person to person via unprotected sex, from needles contaminated with infected blood, through blood transfusion or organ donation from people with the virus, and from mother to baby.

AIDS (Acquired Immune Deficiency Syndrome) is diagnosed when the immune system has been weakened so much by HIV that it can't fight certain life-threatening infections and illnesses.

Worldwide figures estimate that over 40 million people are living with HIV and around three million people die each year from AIDS-related illnesses.

HIV in the UK

The number of people living with HIV in the UK has increased steadily since the 1980s when the virus was discovered. Official figures for 2005 put this at nearly 63,500 people.

Most HIV infections in the UK occur in homosexual men. Transmission of the virus through heterosexual contact has significantly increased in recent years. However, the majority of these infections are in people who have come to live in the UK from countries where HIV is widespread and have been diagnosed since living in the UK.

HIV and the immune system

The immune system protects your body against infection. A key part is white blood cells. These cells find and destroy invading germs, such as bacteria and viruses, preventing the development of serious diseases and damage to your body. HIV avoids being destroyed by the immune system by repeatedly changing its outer 'coat'. It multiplies (replicates) within the special type of white blood cells called CD4 cells. These cells are normally involved in helping other types of immune cell to attack and destroy disease-causing germs.

As HIV multiplies, it destroys CD4 cells, so there are less of them. The reduction in CD4 cells means that the body's ability to fight infection is weakened.

Causes

HIV can only be passed to someone else when the levels of the virus are high enough in the blood or other body fluids and are passed to another person.

HIV infection can be passed via blood, semen, breast milk and vaginal fluids. Therefore, you can pass or have HIV passed to you during unprotected anal or vaginal sex.

There is a small chance of infection through unprotected oral sex. It's estimated around three in every 100 homosexual men with HIV get it through unprotected oral sex with a man who has HIV. The risk of oral transmission from women is extremely low.

The virus can be passed from mother to baby if she has HIV during pregnancy, childbirth or when breastfeeding. HIV can also be passed on if you use infected needles for injections, piercings or tattoos.

HIV is not found in high enough levels in other body fluids such as saliva, sweat, urine or on the skin to cause an infection from contact with these fluids.

HIV can't be passed on through normal day-to-day activities, such as sharing cutlery, sitting on toilet seats or by shaking hands.

HIV and blood or organ donation

In the past, people have become infected with HIV through blood or organ donations. All donations in the UK are now screened for HIV, so the chances of this happening are extremely low.

Symptoms

The period immediately after a person becomes infected with HIV is called primary HIV infection. At this point you are very infectious because the level of the virus will be high in the blood. You will have symptoms of

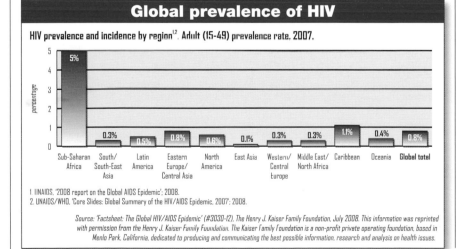

Global prevalence of HIV

HIV prevalence and incidence by region[1,2]. Adult (15-49) prevalence rate, 2007.

Region	Percentage
Sub-Saharan Africa	5%
South/South-East Asia	0.3%
Latin America	0.5%
Eastern Europe/Central Asia	0.8%
North America	0.6%
East Asia	0.1%
Western/Central Europe	0.3%
Middle East/North Africa	0.3%
Caribbean	1.1%
Oceania	0.4%
Global total	0.8%

1. UNAIDS, '2008 report on the Global AIDS Epidemic', 2008.
2. UNAIDS/WHO, 'Core Slides: Global Summary of the HIV/AIDS Epidemic, 2007', 2008.

Source: 'Factsheet: The Global HIV/AIDS Epidemic' (#3030-12), The Henry J. Kaiser Family Foundation, July 2008. This information was reprinted with permission from the Henry J. Kaiser Family Foundation. The Kaiser Family Foundation is a non-profit private operating foundation, based in Menlo Park, California, dedicated to producing and communicating the best possible information, research and analysis on health issues.

HIV infection but you may miss them because they are like other infections such as flu. Early symptoms usually start about two to six weeks after the infection and last approximately five to 10 days. Some symptoms may last longer.

Signs of primary HIV include:
⇨ fever
⇨ swollen glands
⇨ sore throat
⇨ rash on the body or face
⇨ painful muscles or joints
⇨ headache
⇨ feeling sick and vomiting
⇨ ulcers on the mouth, genitals and oesophagus (tube that goes to the stomach).

More serious symptoms include heavy bleeding if you are injured. Rarely, brain infections such as meningitis can affect people with HIV infection.

Worldwide figures estimate that over 40 million people are living with HIV and around three million people die each year from AIDS-related illnesses

---

After the early symptoms, HIV may remain undetected for a number of years until your body's ability to fight infections is reduced. When this happens the number of cells which fight infections has decreased so much that your immune system can't function properly. This leaves the body vulnerable to infections. If a person develops certain life-threatening illnesses it is known as AIDS or advanced HIV disease.

AIDS
Once the immune system has been damaged, infections appear. Common infections include a type of pneumonia called pneumocystis, and tuberculosis.

Other AIDS-related illnesses can include:
⇨ various cancers
⇨ fungal, bacterial or viral infections

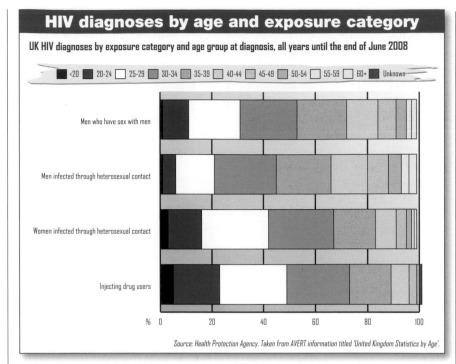

HIV diagnoses by age and exposure category

UK HIV diagnoses by exposure category and age group at diagnosis, all years until the end of June 2008

Legend: ■ <20 ■ 20-24 ☐ 25-29 ■ 30-34 ■ 35-39 ☐ 40-44 ☐ 45-49 ■ 50-54 ☐ 55-59 ☐ 60+ ■ Unknown

Categories: Men who have sex with men; Men infected through heterosexual contact; Women infected through heterosexual contact; Injecting drug users

% 0   20   40   60   80   100

Source: Health Protection Agency. Taken from AVERT information titled 'United Kingdom Statistics by Age'.

⇨ sight problems
⇨ dementia.

Diagnosis

It's important to have an HIV test if you think you have been at risk of HIV infection. There are powerful and effective treatments that slow the virus. Early diagnosis can help ensure you get the best treatment so you can live a full and active life.

To test for HIV, blood is taken. HIV testing in the laboratory involves looking at a blood sample for HIV antibodies, the body's defence chemicals produced in response to infection. Testing can be done four to six weeks after infection but the virus may not be detected in the blood for up to three months in some people.

Testing is usually carried out at genitourinary medicine (GUM) clinics, where sexually transmitted infections are diagnosed and treated. Sometimes results are available after a week, some clinics offer same-day HIV testing.

Before you have a blood test for HIV you may be able to see a counsellor. The test can be explained and the implications of a possible positive diagnosis discussed. You can also talk about the test results with your GP or a counsellor.

Treatment

There is no cure for HIV infection, but treatment with anti-HIV medicines

dramatically slows the progress of the disease and has significantly reduced the number of deaths caused by AIDS-related illnesses. When used appropriately and taken properly, anti-HIV medicines can mean a person with HIV has a near-normal life expectancy.

HIV treatment is managed by specialist outpatient clinics, staffed by doctors, nurses and other health professionals. The status of your immune system and your general health is reviewed on a regular basis.

Usually, once the number of CD4 white blood cells has fallen to a low level, or if the amount of virus in your blood is very high, your specialist will recommend starting drug treatment. Treatment may be started if you develop a serious infection.

Medication
Current treatments prevent the virus from replicating in the body. This in turn reduces the amount of virus in the blood and allows the immune system to recover. To achieve this, three antiretroviral medicines are usually taken together. They normally have to be taken once a day but some need to be taken up to three times a day and at specific times. This combination therapy is termed highly active antiretroviral therapy (HAART) and has dramatically cut the number of deaths from AIDS-related illnesses since its introduction. There are

three main classes of antiretroviral medicine. Combination therapies usually contain medicines from two of these classes.

Nucleoside reverse transcriptase inhibitors (NRTIs)

NRTIs prevent HIV from copying its genetic information and so multiplying. They include abacavir (e.g. Ziagen), lamivudine (e.g. Zeffix) and zidovudine (e.g. Retrovir).

Protease inhibitors (PIs)

PIs prevent the virus from assembling its protective coat before leaving CD4 cells. Ritonavir-boosted protease inhibitors may be used to increase the potency of the medicine. They include atazanavir (e.g. Reyataz) and saquinavir (e.g. Invirase).

Non-nucleoside reverse transcriptase inhibitors (NNRTIs)

NNRTIs are a highly effective class of antiretrovirals, which have a similar mode of action to NRTIs. They include efavirenz (e.g. Sustiva) and nevirapine (e.g. Viramune).

HIV fusion-inhibitor

An HIV fusion-inhibitor is a medicine used in combination with other medicines when the infection is no longer controlled by other treatments. There is just one fusion-inhibitor, enfuvirtide (Fuzeon).

Potential new treatments

In the future, further anti-HIV medicines may be produced. These may include medicines that stimulate the patient's own immune system to fight off HIV or target the virus in different ways. Integrase inhibitors are a new class of medicine being developed. One example is raltegravir, which is currently in human trials and is showing promise.

CCR5 inhibitors are also in development, one of which is maraviroc and studies of these medicines are continuing.

Second-generation NNRTs such as etravirine have recently been developed but are not widely available yet.

There are also real hopes that a cure for HIV infection and a vaccine to prevent infection will be developed.

Side effects

The combination treatment can cause side effects. In the first few months, you may feel sick, vomit and have a headache, although these often wear off. Some medicines can cause sleep disturbances or depression. PIs and NRTIs are associated with a syndrome called lipodystrophy, which involves a thinning of the face, arms, legs and buttocks, and a build-up of fat on the belly, breasts and back. The redistribution of fat can be managed, for example, by changing the combination treatment and changing your diet and exercise. Lipodystrophy, caused by PIs, can also increase the risk of heart disease.

Prevention

HIV and body fluids

The risk of HIV infection is dramatically reduced by using a condom. Condoms shouldn't be used with an oil-based lubricant, such as petroleum jelly (e.g. Vaseline) or baby oil, because this can cause the latex to break down. Use water-based lubricants (e.g. KY jelly, Sylk) instead; however, remember that condoms don't completely eliminate the risk. Reducing the number of partners reduces overall risk.

HIV and pregnancy

An HIV test is routinely offered to all pregnant women early on in their pregnancy. If you have HIV you can be treated to reduce the risk of transmitting it to your baby. HIV medicines can be taken during pregnancy, delivery and when breastfeeding. Birth by caesarean section may also be needed if the virus is found in the blood. Your baby may be given medicines in the first few weeks of life to prevent infection. If you have HIV you can consider alternatives to breastfeeding to prevent transmission of the virus.

HIV and needlestick injury for healthcare workers

This can be avoided by using single-use or sterilised needles.

Taking medicines by injection

If you inject medicines you shouldn't share injection equipment.

Living with HIV

In countries where HIV treatment is limited, AIDS-related illness is a common cause of death. In the UK, most people with HIV have access to anti-HIV medicines and go on to lead full and active lives.

Further information

⇨ Terrence Higgins Trust
0845 1221 200
www.tht.org.uk
⇨ NAM
020 7840 0050
www.aidsmap.com
January 2008

⇨ Information from Bupa. Visit www.bupa.co.uk for more.
© Bupa

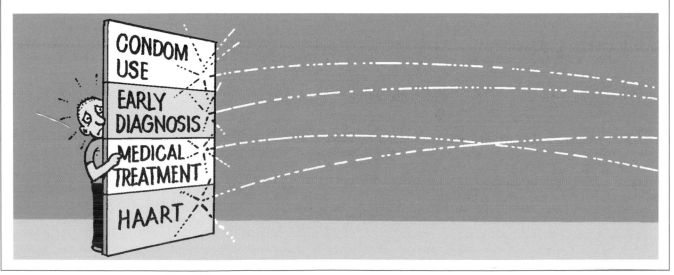

HIV/AIDS estimates are revised downwards

An extract from the World Health Organisation's report *World Health Statistics 2008*

HIV/AIDS is one of the most urgent threats to global public health. Most of the infections with HIV and deaths due to the disease could be prevented if people everywhere had access to good services for preventing and treating HIV infection. Estimates of the size and course of the HIV epidemic are updated every year by UNAIDS and WHO. In 2007, improved survey data and advances in estimation methodologies led to substantially revised estimates of numbers of people living with HIV, of HIV-related deaths and of new infections worldwide.

The number of people living with HIV continues to rise but is lower than previously estimated

The number of people living with HIV worldwide in 2007 was estimated at 33.2 million; there may be as few as 30.6 million or as many as 36.1 million. The latest estimates cannot be compared directly with estimates published in previous years. The new data and improved methods used in 2007 also led to a substantial revision

of the estimates for 2006 and before. For instance, the new best estimate for 2006 is now 32 million and not 39.5 million as published in 2006. For 2000, UNAIDS and WHO now estimate that 27.6 million people were infected, compared with 36.1 million estimated at that time.

Sub-Saharan Africa continues to be the region most affected by HIV/AIDS. In 2007, one in every three people in the world living with HIV lived in sub-Saharan Africa, a total of 22.5 million. Although other regions are less severely affected, 4 million people in south and south-east Asia and 1.6 million in eastern Europe and central Asia were living with HIV/AIDS.

While total numbers of people living with HIV have risen, overall prevalence has not changed

Although the total number of people living with HIV has increased significantly over the years, the proportion infected has not changed since the end of the 1990s. In fact, the number of people who become infected every day (over 6,800)

is greater than the number who die of the disease (around 6,000). Worldwide, 0.8% of the adult population (aged 15–49 years) is estimated to be infected with HIV, with a range of 0.7–0.9%.

Sub-Saharan Africa continues to be the region most affected by HIV/AIDS

In sub-Saharan Africa, the estimated proportion of the population infected has actually fallen steadily since 2000. Current data indicate that HIV prevalence reached a peak of nearly 6% around 2000 and fell to about 5% in 2007. This reflects significant changes in high-risk forms of behaviour in a number of countries but is also a result of the maturity of the pandemic, especially in sub-Saharan Africa where HIV first took hold among the general population.

Understanding the data and estimates

HIV infection is detected by testing for HIV antibodies in the blood, although in practice only a small proportion of people ever have an HIV test. This is particularly true in developing countries, where access to health care services is limited. For many years, scientists trying to estimate HIV prevalence had to rely on tests carried out on the blood of pregnant women attending antenatal care in clinics equipped to test for HIV. There are many problems in relying on this approach. Not all women attend for antenatal care and not all antenatal clinics have the ability to test for HIV, although in some cases tests are done at central

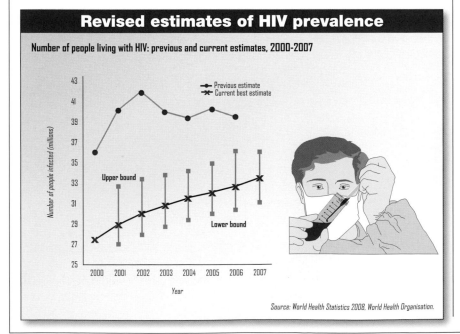

Revised estimates of HIV prevalence

Number of people living with HIV: previous and current estimates, 2000-2007

Source: World Health Statistics 2008, World Health Organisation.

level. In general, both antenatal care attendance and availability of antibody testing are higher in urban than in rural areas. In addition, bias can arise because pregnant women are not representative of the population at risk of HIV infection, especially in settings where HIV is largely confined to high-risk groups such as sex workers or men who have sex with men. In some settings, HIV testing of groups at high risk of infection has been used to estimate overall prevalence, but these estimates will be accurate only if infection outside the high-risk groups is low.

More recently, it has been possible to introduce antibody testing into household surveys that have large samples of the population selected at random. This gives a more unbiased estimate of the overall prevalence of HIV infection, provided survey participation rates are high. Since 2001, 30 countries in sub-Saharan Africa, Asia and the Caribbean have included HIV testing in household surveys. It was found that prevalence estimates from surveys are generally lower than those calculated on the basis of pregnant women or high-risk groups. The most dramatic example of this was in India: in the National Family Health Survey, 100,000 adults from all over the country were tested for HIV and 0.28% were found to be infected, half the level generated by the earlier methods. This has resulted in a significantly lower estimate of the number of people living with HIV in India. Overall, 70% of the downward adjustment in 2007 is accounted for by new figures for just six countries: Angola, India, Kenya, Mozambique, Nigeria and Zimbabwe.

There have also been improvements to the methods used for estimating HIV prevalence in countries without survey-based data. For example, it is now clear that pregnant women attending antenatal clinics in major cities are more likely to be infected with HIV than adults in general. Therefore, reliance on testing women in urban antenatal clinics tends to overestimate the prevalence of HIV. The new estimates have been adjusted to reflect this.

Estimating mortality due to AIDS is difficult in developing countries, where most deaths occur but where systems for counting deaths and recording cause of death are weak or nonexistent.

Currently, new infection rates and deaths due to HIV/AIDS are estimated from the application of statistical models using data on HIV prevalence, average time between HIV infection and death in the absence of treatment, and survival rates of people receiving treatment. In the absence of antiretroviral treatment, the net median survival time after infection with HIV is now estimated to be 11 years, instead of the previously estimated 9 years. These changes are based on recent information generated by longitudinal research studies. For the same level of prevalence, this longer average survival period has resulted in lower estimates of new infections and deaths due to AIDS.

The contribution of the number of people on antiretroviral treatment to the total number of people living with HIV/AIDS is still small. In the future, however, as more people benefit from treatment and live longer with HIV infection, this will increasingly affect the number of people in the world living with HIV/AIDS.

⇨ The above information is reprinted with kind permission from the World Health Organisation. Visit www.who.int for more information.
© *World Health Organisation*

Gender inequalities and HIV

Information from the World Health Organisation

According to the latest (2008) WHO and UNAIDS global estimates, women comprise 50% of people living with HIV.

In sub-Saharan Africa, women constitute 60% of people living with HIV. In other regions, men having sex with men (MSM), injecting drug users (IDU), sex workers and their clients are among those most at risk for HIV, but the proportion of women living with HIV has been increasing in the last 10 years.

This includes married or regular partners of clients of commercial sex, IDU and MSM, as well as female sex workers and injecting drug users.

Gender inequalities are a key driver of the epidemic in several ways:

Gender norms related to masculinity can encourage men to have more sexual partners and older men to have sexual relations with much younger women.

In some settings, this contributes to higher infection rates among young women (15-24 years) compared to young men.

Norms related to masculinity, i.e. homophobia, stigmatises men having sex with men, and makes them and their partners vulnerable to HIV.

Norms related to femininity can prevent women – especially young women – from accessing HIV information and services. Only 38% of young women have accurate, comprehensive knowledge of HIV/AIDS according to the 2008 UNAIDS global figures.

HIV/AIDS programmes can address harmful gender norms and stereotypes including by working with men and boys to change norms related to fatherhood, sexual responsibility, decision-making and violence, and by providing comprehensive, age-appropriate HIV/AIDS education for young people that addresses gender norms.

Violence against women (physical, sexual and emotional), which is experienced by 10 to 60% of women (ages 15-49 years) worldwide, increases their vulnerability to HIV.

Forced sex can contribute to HIV transmission due to tears and lacerations resulting from the use of force.

Women who fear or experience violence lack the power to ask their partners to use condoms or refuse unprotected sex. Fear of violence can prevent women from learning and/or sharing their HIV status and accessing treatment.

Programmes can address violence against women by offering safer sex negotiation and life skills training, helping women who fear or experience violence to safely disclose their HIV status, providing comprehensive medico-legal services to victims of sexual violence, and working with countries to develop, strengthen and enforce laws that eliminate violence against women.

Gender-related barriers in access to services prevent women and men from accessing HIV prevention, treatment and care.

Women may face barriers due to their lack of access to and control over resources, child-care responsibilities, restricted mobility and limited decision-making power.

Socialisation of men may mean that they will not seek HIV services due to a fear of stigma and discrimination, losing their jobs and of being perceived as 'weak' or 'unmanly'.

Programmes can improve access to services for women and men by removing financial barriers in access to services, bringing services closer to the community, and addressing HIV-related stigma and discrimination, including in health care settings.

Women assume the major share of care-giving in the family, including for those living with and affected by HIV. This is often unpaid and is based on the assumption that women 'naturally' fill this role.

Programmes can support women in their care-giving roles by offering community-based care and support, including by increasing men's involvement.

Lack of education and economic security affects millions of women and girls, whose literacy levels are generally lower than men and boys'.

Many women, especially those living with HIV, lose their homes, inheritance, possessions, livelihoods and even their children when their partners die. This forces many women to adopt survival strategies that increase their chances of contracting and spreading HIV. Educating girls makes them more equipped to make safer sexual decisions.

Programmes can promote economic opportunities for women (e.g. through microfinance and micro-credit, vocational and skills training and other income generation activities), protect and promote their inheritance rights, and expand efforts to keep girls in school.

Many national HIV/AIDS programmes fail to address underlying gender inequalities. In 2008, only 52% of countries who reported to the UN General Assembly included specific, budgeted support for women-focused HIV/AIDS programmes.

HIV/AIDS programmes should collect and use sex and age disaggregated data to monitor and evaluate impact of programmes on different populations, build capacity of key stakeholders to address gender inequalities, facilitate meaningful participation of women's groups, women living with HIV and young people, and allocate resources for programme elements that address gender inequalities.

⇨ The above information is reprinted with kind permission from the World Health Organisation. Visit www.who.int for more information.
© *World Health Organisation*

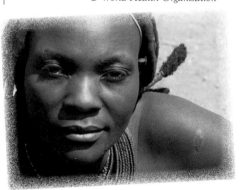

Protect the children

Information from the Global AIDS Alliance

Did you know?

HIV/AIDS is having a staggering impact on children. Worldwide, over 15 million children under the age of 18 have lost one or both parents to AIDS – a number that is expected to reach 20 million by 2010. In sub-Saharan Africa, 12 million children – 80% of the global total – have been orphaned by AIDS, and millions more live in households where an adult is sick.

Studies have found that orphans are more likely to be stunted in their growth and less likely to attend school than children living with both parents. Poor nutrition and limited access to health services put orphans at increased risk of starvation, illness, and death. And without nurturing from a loving parent or guardian, children's emotional development is often diminished, too.

Many AIDS orphans are themselves infected with HIV, and worldwide at least two million children under the age of 15 are living with HIV/AIDS. Another 1,000 children are newly infected with HIV each day – most through mother-to-child transmission of the virus. Worldwide, over 270,000 children die of AIDS each year, and in some countries the epidemic accounts for as many as half of all deaths among children under five.

All told, children under the age of 15 account for 14% of both AIDS-related deaths and new HIV infections worldwide. But only 6% of the approximately three million people now on treatment are children. And only 33% of HIV-positive pregnant women are receiving antiretroviral medications that can virtually eliminate mother-to-child transmission of the virus. Antiretrovirals formulated to treat children with AIDS can cost five times as much as adult formulations, and pediatric doses are not widely available. In addition, the expensive and complicated tests required to diagnose paediatric HIV mean that half of HIV-infected children die undiagnosed before their second birthday.

Worldwide, over 15 million children under the age of 18 have lost one or both parents to AIDS – a number that is expected to reach 20 million by 2010

HIV/AIDS is exacerbating the desperate situation of children worldwide. As the epidemic kills more and more adults, the traditional safety net for orphans and other vulnerable children – the extended family – is stretched to the breaking point. Fewer resources are available for basic health, education, and nutrition services. In households where adults are living with AIDS, older children are often responsible for supporting their families and providing care. Children living in child-headed households, on the street, or with families who regard them as an unwanted burden are particularly vulnerable to neglect, abuse, and exploitation. And those subjected to abuse or exploitation are at increased risk of HIV infection. Children of all ages struggle with the pain of losing a parent and the stigma of living in a family touched by HIV/AIDS. Even children who are spared a family bereavement often lose their teachers, doctors, neighbours, and other adult role models to HIV/AIDS.

Despite their vulnerability, children have been largely overlooked in the response to HIV. According to UNICEF, less than 10% of children orphaned and made vulnerable by HIV/AIDS receive any public support or services. And just one in seven of the estimated 780,000 children in urgent need of antiretroviral therapy are receiving treatment.

What needs to be done?

The critical first step in slowing the paediatric AIDS epidemic is

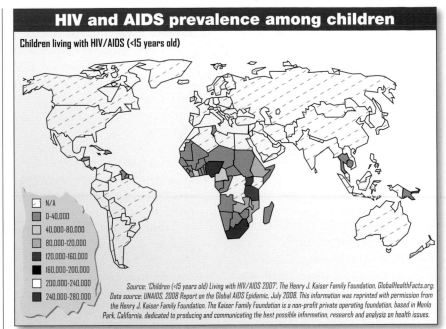

HIV and AIDS prevalence among children

Children living with HIV/AIDS (<15 years old)

- N/A
- 0-40,000
- 40,000-80,000
- 80,000-120,000
- 120,000-160,000
- 160,000-200,000
- 200,000-240,000
- 240,000-280,000

Source: 'Children (<15 years old) Living with HIV/AIDS 2007', The Henry J. Kaiser Family Foundation, GlobalHealthFacts.org; Data source: UNAIDS, 2008 Report on the Global AIDS Epidemic, July 2008. This information was reprinted with permission from the Henry J. Kaiser Family Foundation. The Kaiser Family Foundation is a non-profit private operating foundation, based in Menlo Park, California, dedicated to producing and communicating the best possible information, research and analysis on health issues.

to prevent HIV transmission from pregnant mothers to their babies, and governments, multilateral agencies, service delivery organisations, and pharmaceutical companies must do more to scale up prevention of mother-to-child transmission (PMTCT) programmes. In addition, while there has been important progress in expanding the number of paediatric treatments, there remains a lack of diagnostic tools for infants younger than 18 months.

Orphans and vulnerable children (OVC), including children with HIV/AIDS, need comprehensive care and support. This includes access to education, health care, shelter, food and nutrition, and psychosocial support. Orphans and vulnerable children also need special protection against abuse, violence, exploitation, discrimination, trafficking, and loss of inheritance. Providing treatment and care to parents with HIV/AIDS will help keep families intact as long as possible, and, of course, children with HIV must receive treatment.

In addition, families and local communities need help so they can raise orphans and vulnerable children in a supportive non-institutional environment. Indeed, many experts believe that strengthening community-based efforts is the only hope for building effective, sustainable support systems for orphans and other vulnerable children.

Finally, all children must have access to a free, quality basic education,

and all children must be protected against violence that threatens their physical and emotional well-being and increases their risk of HIV infection.

Here are just a few examples of programmes that are making a difference:

⇨ In Rwanda, a community-based project provides livestock and other income-generation assistance to AIDS orphans, and trains *nkundabanas*, adults in the community who can mentor and support orphaned children.

⇨ In Zambia's Eastern Province, local nonprofits successfully lobbied to exempt orphans and vulnerable children from having to pay school fees.

⇨ In Mombasa, Kenya, a family care clinic is providing free ARV medications and other support services to children living with AIDS.

⇨ In Turkmenistan, a life-skills training programme is teaching students how HIV is transmitted and how they can protect themselves – and encouraging them to educate others.

⇨ Across Africa, local health clinics provide children with cotrimoxazole, an inexpensive antibiotic that prevents potentially fatal infections in HIV-positive children and can also delay the onset of AIDS and the need for ARV treatment.

⇨ In Malawi and Ghana, a pilot

programme is improving school safety by making curriculum reforms, training teachers and other school staff, and making important infrastructure changes such as building separate latrines for boys and girls.

Programmes like these help show us the way forward. But they must be scaled up dramatically in order to address the growing crisis of orphans and vulnerable children.

What is the Global AIDS Alliance doing?

The Global AIDS Alliance is working to mobilise the political will and financial resources needed to ensure comprehensive care and support for orphans and vulnerable children, including children affected by HIV/AIDS. In particular, we are working to achieve the following goals:

⇨ Scale up prevention of mother-to-child HIV transmission programmes, with the goal of ensuring that 80% of pregnant HIV-infected women have access to PMTCT services.

⇨ Increase effective diagnosis and treatment of paediatric AIDS, with the goal of ensuring that at least 15% of those receiving ARV therapy are children under the age of 15.

⇨ Ensure effective implementation of US legislation that mandates comprehensive care and support for OVC, including food and nutrition, psychosocial services, protection of inheritance rights, paediatric AIDS treatment, and school fee abolition.

⇨ Secure increased funding for OVC programmes in poor countries and ensure that the US allocates at least 10% of its global AIDS funding to OVC programmes.

⇨ Accelerate universal basic education and the abolition of school fees.

⇨ Advance a comprehensive response to violence against children, with a focus on reducing girls' vulnerability to HIV and making schools safe.

These efforts will help ensure that all children have access to essential health, basic education, food and nutrition, psychosocial support, and other services. In addition, addressing the needs of orphans and vulnerable children will encourage long-term economic growth in poor countries hardest hit by HIV and bolster social and political stability. Ultimately, ensuring comprehensive care and support for OVC will encourage progress toward the Millennium Development Goals of achieving universal basic education (MDG #2), reducing child mortality (MDG #4), and combating HIV/AIDS, malaria, and other diseases (MDG #6).

⇨ The above information is reprinted with kind permission from the Global AIDS Alliance. Visit www.globalaidsalliance.org for more information.

© Global AIDS Alliance

Life expectancy of HIV patients increases

Information from the University of Bristol

HIV-infected patients in high income countries are living some 13 years longer thanks to improvements in combination antiretroviral therapy (cART), according to new research by the University of Bristol published in an HIV Special Issue of *The Lancet* today.

Improvements in and long-term effectiveness of cART have seen life expectancy increase by some 13 years from 1996-99 to 2003-05, and an accompanying drop in mortality of nearly 40 per cent in the same period.

However, life expectancy in these patients remains well short of the general population, and patients treated late in the course of their infection have worse life expectancy.

Since cART was introduced in 1996, combination therapy regimens have become more effective, better tolerated, and have been simplified in terms of dosing. However, the effect of HIV on life expectancy in the era of combination therapy is not well understood due to the relative novelty of this treatment.

Professor Jonathan Sterne of Bristol University's Department of Social Medicine and Professor Robert Hogg of British Columbia Centre for Excellence in HIV/AIDS and Simon Fraser University, Vancouver, Canada and colleagues from the Antiretroviral Therapy Cohort Collaboration (ART-CC) compared changes in mortality and life expectancy among HIV-positive individuals on cART.

This collaboration of 14 studies in Europe and North America analysed 18,587; 13,914, and 10,584 patients who started cART in 1996-99, 2000-02, and 2003-05 respectively.

A total of 2,056 patients died during the study period, with mortality decreasing from 16.3 deaths per 1000 person-years in 1996-99 to 10.0 in 2003-05 – a drop of around 40 per cent.

Potential life years lost per 1000 person-years also decreased over the same time, from 366 to 189 – a fall of 48 per cent. Life expectancy increased from 36.1 years in 1996-99 to 49.4 years in 2003-05, an increase of more than 13 years.

Patients treated later in the course of their infection, with lower CD4+ cell counts (below 100 cells per µl blood at initiation of cART), had shorter life expectancy, at 32.4 years, compared with 50.4 years in patients treated at earlier stages with higher CD4 loads (above 200 cells per µl).

Patients with presumed transmission via injecting drug use had a shorter life expectancy (32.6 years) than those from other transmission groups (44.7 years). Finally, women had a slightly longer life expectancy than men (44.2 v 42.8 years), which may be due to women on average starting their treatment earlier in the course of HIV-infection.

Despite these positive results, an HIV-positive person starting cART at age 20 will only, on average, live another 43 years (to age 63), while a 20- year-old HIV-negative person in a high-income country can expect to live to around 80 years, a difference of nearly 20 years. This last finding leads the authors to call on health planners to improve health services and living conditions for HIV-infected patients to reduce this gap.

Professor Sterne said: 'The progressive reductions in mortality and gains in life expectancy over the three periods studied here are probably the result of both improvements in therapy during the first decade of cART and continuing declines in mortality rates among individuals on such treatment for long periods.

'These advances have transformed HIV from being a fatal disease, which was the reality for patients before the advent of combination treatment, into a long-term chronic condition.

'The results of this study indicate that people living with HIV in high-income countries can expect increasing positive health outcomes on cART. The marked increase in life expectancy since 1996 is a testament to the gradual improvement and overall success of such treatment.'

Further information

Paper: 'Life expectancy of individuals on combination antiretroviral therapy in high-income countries: a collaborative analysis of 14 cohort studies' by The Antiretroviral Therapy Cohort Collaboration. *Lancet* 2008; 372: 293–99
25 July 2008

⇨ The above information is reprinted with kind permission from the University of Bristol. Visit www.bristol.ac.uk for more information.
© *University of Bristol*

Gay men with HIV have near-normal death rates

Information from Positive Nation

A study of HIV patients in 24 countries by the UK Medical Research Council has found that gay men who don't allow their CD4 counts to drop below 350 now have near-normal death rates compared to the general population, even off treatment.

The study of nearly 47,500 patients in HIV clinics in the UK, the USA, Germany, Switzerland and Belgium, found that gay men in this category only had a 20% higher death rate than other men in the same country and of similar age.

However, the same study found that people who had caught HIV through heterosexual sex were still over three times more likely to die, and people who were (or had been) injecting drug users were ten times more likely, probably due to the influence of co-infections like hepatitis C.

The study looked at patients who registered at least one CD4 count of 350 while off HIV drugs and monitored their death rates until they started treatment or died. Half of the group were gay men and about a quarter each heterosexuals and injecting drug users.

It found a total of 426 deaths in this population. Comparing these to expected death rates, it found 117 deaths in gay men where 97 would have been expected in the general population; 82 compared with 24 in heterosexuals; and 227 compared with 22 in injecting drug users. Women were about 25% less likely to die than men. The death rate went up as people aged with people in their fifties three times more likely to die and people in their sixties six times.

However, the finding that, even off-treatment, a significant group of people have the potential to live near-normal lifespans can only be good news.
March 2008

⇨ The above information is reprinted with kind permission from Positive Nation. Visit www.positivenation.co.uk for more information.
© *Sugar media*

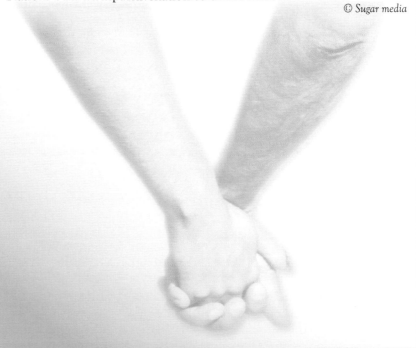

HIV in developing countries

Frequently asked questions

Doesn't everyone know about it already?

If there's so much AIDS in developing countries, everyone over there must know about it. So why is it still spreading? Millions of people around the world have no access to reliable healthcare information and often do not hear about HIV and AIDS until it is too late. Also, knowing information is only a small part of changing behaviour (ask any smoker you know!). To understand the spread of the virus, we need to understand the realities of life in poor countries.

Poverty is one of the major causes of the spread of HIV

Doesn't everyone know to use a condom?

When will people stop having unsafe sex? Surely everyone knows to use a condom now? 'After I became ill and tested HIV positive I discovered that both my husband and his family knew that he had HIV before we were married.' This woman from Kousalya, India, is not alone in this experience.

Preventing HIV is more complex than simply the need to use condoms. For example, in many parts of the world the number of children couples have measures their status in the community. Everyone has the right to choose whether to have children or not – and everyone knows it is not possible to have children while using condoms.

It is also estimated that even in the United States, where access to information, testing and treatment is good, 25% of people with HIV do not know they are HIV positive. This number is very significantly higher in developing countries.

Why is HIV such a problem in poor countries?

Why is HIV such a problem in poor countries? Poverty is one of the major causes of the spread of HIV and of people's health decline to AIDS. Fighting HIV and AIDS in societies where the priority is finding enough food for the family each day will always be difficult.

Poor people in developing countries are often faced with difficult choices such as going hungry that night, or making money in whatever way possible to put food on the table. Often this involves selling sex and so increasing risk to HIV.

While the first choice involves immediate and definite risks (hunger), the second involves only possible risk (HIV infection). Even in countries where HIV rates are as high as 39%, there is still a 61% chance of not becoming infected. And even if one does become infected, it is often some years before illness and debilitation set in. It is a risk some have no choice but to take.

Why is there stigma around HIV and AIDS, if so many people are affected?

How can there be stigma around HIV and AIDS in developing countries when so many people are affected? We all know that stigma surrounds HIV and AIDS, but there is a common belief that there is less stigma about HIV and AIDS in developing countries because so many people are affected. This is not the case. Societies everywhere are underpinned by accepted and unaccepted norms, values and behaviours – often relating to sex. In many African countries, for instance, AIDS widows are ousted from their homes and communities because, even though it is commonly accepted that men can have several wives and partners, the wives are almost always blamed for their husbands' HIV infection. Prejudice and fear prevail and with fewer safety-nets such as government welfare support and women's shelters, women and children in particular (often HIV positive themselves) find they are left with no money, home or belongings and without the skills to find work.

Anyone living with HIV in a developing country will tell you that the stigma applies everywhere, and people often conceal having HIV for safety reasons. All over the world the association of HIV with sexual behaviour, illness and death and specifically with highly stigmatised issues such as homosexuality and drug use means that fighting HIV is more difficult. ActionAid works to challenge the stigma and prejudice that surround HIV and AIDS.

How does AIDS in developing countries affect me?

All these countries are so far away – AIDS over there doesn't affect me. AIDS is having such a devastating effect on the workforce of so many countries that the ripples are being felt all over our increasingly globalised world. Economically speaking, lost people equal lost markets and lost profit. But more importantly, morally our ultimate aim should be lives free from unnecessary suffering. HIV and AIDS is a preventable and manageable condition. We all have a responsibility to save suffering and lives, and our governments – who answer directly to us – play a huge part in helping to make this a reality.

'If AIDS doesn't get them, something else will'

If so many people in developing countries have HIV and AIDS they must be used to dealing with it by now, and anyway, if AIDS doesn't get them something else will. People should never have to get used to dealing with pain, tragedy and illness. HIV and AIDS decimate communities and lives and although those affected do find solutions and ways of coping, there is so much that could be done at the international level. Everybody has the right to a healthy life, and it is the responsibility of us all to help others around the world to achieve this.

⇨ Reproduced by kind permission of ActionAid International. For more information on this and related topics, please visit the ActionAid website at www.actionaid.org.uk

What do you know about HIV/AIDS?

Use this quiz to test your knowledge about HIV/AIDS

1. HIV/AIDS is a disease which mainly affects gay people.
- [ ] true
- [ ] false

2. HIV/AIDS is a fatal disease.
- [ ] true
- [ ] false

3. You can catch HIV/AIDS by sharing a drinking glass with an infected person.
- [ ] true
- [ ] false

4. Mothers can pass HIV/AIDS on to their babies during pregnancy, birth and breastfeeding.
- [ ] true
- [ ] false

5. Having sex with someone infected with HIV/AIDS is the only way you can get HIV/AIDS.
- [ ] true
- [ ] false

6. HIV/AIDS is only a problem in the developing world.
- [ ] true
- [ ] false

7. Using a condom reduces the chances of you becoming infected with HIV/AIDS.
- [ ] true
- [ ] false

8. HIV/AIDS can now be cured.
- [ ] true
- [ ] false

Answers

1. HIV/AIDS is a disease which mainly affects gay people.
This statement is **false**. AIDS was first discovered among the gay community in the USA but worldwide it affects anyone and everyone. More people have been infected with HIV/AIDS by heterosexual sex than by any other method of transmission.

2. HIV/AIDS is a fatal disease.
This statement is **true**. HIV/AIDS eventually destroys the body's immune system. Eventually anyone infected with HIV will die of AIDS itself or of the other diseases which they get as a result of their damaged immune system.

3. You can catch HIV/AIDS by sharing a drinking glass with an infected person.
This statement is **false**. The human immunodeficiency virus (HIV) does not survive for any length of time outside the human body. You cannot catch HIV/AIDS by sharing drinking glasses, using the same toilets or touching a person infected with HIV/AIDS.

4. Mothers can pass HIV/AIDS on to their babies during pregnancy, birth and breastfeeding.
This statement is **true**. Women who have HIV/AIDS can pass the virus on to their children before or during birth. Even if the baby is born healthy, it may be infected during the time it is being breastfed, as the virus is found in the mother's milk.

5. Having sex with someone infected with HIV/AIDS is the only way you can get HIV/AIDS.
This statement is **false**. Drug users who share needles, people who are given blood transfusions or blood products in countries where the blood has not been not screened, and babies born to infected women can all be infected with HIV/AIDS.

6. HIV/AIDS is only a problem in the developing world.
This statement is **false**. Although the great majority of people infected with HIV/AIDS live in the developing world, HIV/AIDS is a problem everywhere, including the UK – around 700-900 people die of HIV/AIDS each year in the UK alone.

7. Using a condom reduces the chances of you becoming infected with HIV/AIDS.
This statement is **true**. Safe sex using a condom is one of the most effective ways of preventing the spread of HIV/AIDS between sexual partners.

8. HIV/AIDS can now be cured.
This statement is **false**. Although treatments are much better than they were, and there are drugs which can delay the onset of full-blown AIDS for many years, there are still no drugs which can cure HIV/AIDS or vaccines which can protect people against it.

⇨ The above information is reprinted with kind permission from Pfizer. Visit www.abouthivaids.org for more information

© Pfizer

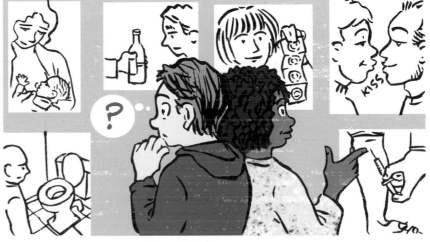

Criminal transmission of HIV

Information from AVERT

For the vast majority of people living with HIV, preventing others from becoming infected with the virus that they carry is a primary concern. HIV positive individuals are, after all, only too aware of just how difficult it can be to live with the illness, and few would wish it on anybody else.

This said, not all HIV+ people take the precautions that they perhaps should. Scare stories of people 'deliberately' or 'recklessly' transmitting HIV to others have appeared in the media since the epidemic first began, and some of the individuals concerned have even been criminally charged and imprisoned for their actions. But while at first it might seem obvious to prosecute someone for recklessly or intentionally infecting another with an ultimately fatal virus, this assumption, and its consequences, can present numerous problems. So what are the issues that must be addressed when prosecuting someone for transmitting HIV? Is it right to try and criminalise HIV+ people in this way? And what can past cases teach us?

Intentional, reckless or accidental?

Before looking at the complexities of prosecuting people for infecting others with HIV, it is first necessary to understand the different types of transmission that can take place. The definitions below are based on general categories and are not specific to any particular country or legal system.

Intentional

Intentional (or deliberate or wilful) transmission, is considered the most serious form of criminal transmission. Some cases have involved individuals (both HIV+ and HIV-) who have used needles or other implements to intentionally infect others with HIV. Others have been based on HIV+ people who have had sex with the primary intent of transmitting the virus to their partner.

Intentional transmission also sometimes takes place when a negative partner has an active desire to become infected with HIV (a practice sometimes referred to as 'sexual thrill seeking' or 'bug chasing'). This is unlikely to lead to prosecution, however, as both parties consent.

Reckless

This is where HIV is transmitted through a careless rather than deliberate act. If for example a person who knows they have HIV has unprotected sex with a negative person, but fails to inform them of the risk involved, this could be classed as reckless transmission in court. 'Reckless' here implies that transmission took place as part of the pursuit of sexual gratification rather than because the HIV+ person intended to give their partner HIV (HIV is of course not 'automatically' transmitted every time someone has unprotected sex.)

Accidental

This is the most common way that HIV is passed on. A person is generally said to have accidentally transmitted HIV if:

⇨ They were unaware that they had the virus, and therefore did not feel the need to take measures to protect their partner.

⇨ They were aware of their HIV+ status and they used a condom during sex, but the condom failed in some way (although there is some debate over whether this should in fact be classed as a reckless act, as we shall see later).

The complexities of prosecution

Unfortunately deciding if someone has intentionally, recklessly or accidentally transmitted HIV is not as simple as the explanations above may suggest. The divisions between each of the three categories can be very blurred, and depend largely on individual interpretation. Even after a decision has been made on what grounds to prosecute, a court may still have a hard time deciding whether to find someone guilty or not. Some of the most problematic issues include:

Proof

It might appear that proof is a straightforward issue, but proving that an individual has transmitted HIV can be exceedingly difficult.

Firstly it needs to be proven that the accused (let's call them A) was definitely the source of the accuser's (B) HIV. This would involve a range of evidence including sexual history, testing history and scientific evidence in the form of phylogenetics. This compares the DNA of the virus that A and B are infected with. If they are completely different then it means B

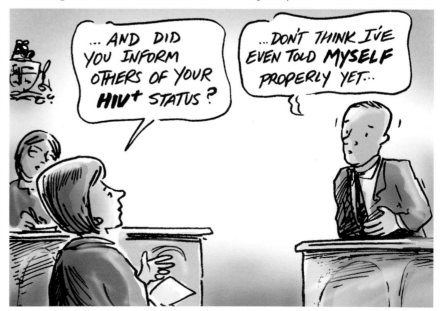

almost certainly did not acquire HIV from A, and the case would probably be thrown out. If the strains are very similar, however, it is possible, though not conclusive, that A infected B. Phylogenetics can not reliably estimate the direction of transmission and therefore it is possible that B infected A. Furthermore, both could have been infected by the same third party, or different third parties who shared similar strains of HIV. Due to its shortcomings, advocates recommend phylogenetic evidence should only be considered in the context of all other evidence.

Often, the only definitive proof would be a negative test on B that was performed after A received a positive test. Even so, if the complainant had had multiple sexual partners, pinning responsibility on a particular individual could be very difficult.

In cases where intentional transmission needs to be proven, evidence needs to be found that A actively intended and wanted to infect B. Unless there is physical proof of this (e.g. a syringe filled with HIV+ material, a note, or a written confession), it can often just be one person's word against another. With cases of sexual transmission, proving intention can be virtually impossible as the very nature of sexual HIV transmission means there are no witnesses: what happens in the bedroom is essentially private. If no evidence of intentional transmission could be found, therefore, a charge of reckless or careless transmission would probably be chosen. Whether someone can be legally charged with reckless (as opposed to intentional) transmission depends entirely on an individual country's laws and courts. In some places there is no differentiation between the two.

Consent and disclosure

Almost all criminal convictions involving sexual transmission are brought about because an HIV+ person has failed to inform their negative partner about their status. In some cases, the positive person may have actively lied in response to a direct question in order to persuade their partner to have unprotected sex. In others, they may simply not have mentioned their condition. A prosecution involving deception might carry a more severe penalty than a simple failure to disclose, because it affects a person's choice to consent to sex. But again, this depends on local laws.

Some say that sex with a condom, but without disclosure of status should also count as reckless transmission.

Scare stories of people 'deliberately' or 'recklessly' transmitting HIV to others have appeared in the media since the epidemic first began

---

Consent is an important issue in all criminal prosecutions. If the accused had simply not mentioned they are HIV+, then the prosecution would probably argue that they had been reckless by not disclosing their status and not informing their partner of the risks involved in intercourse. However, the defence could well counter this by saying that the balance of responsibility is 50:50, and that by agreeing to have unprotected sex, the 'victim' effectively consented to all the risks involved, including that of HIV. This argument was used in the appeal trial of Mohammed Dica, the first person in England to be accused of recklessly transmitting HIV.

If the accused had actively deceived their partner, and told them they were negative when they were not, then the prosecution could quite easily argue that the 50:50 balance of responsibility had been taken away, making the accused more liable to prosecution.

The argument that non-disclosure equals guilt could potentially even be applied if the person on trial had used a condom. Some say that sex with a condom, but without disclosure of status, should also count as reckless transmission. This is because condoms are not always 100% effective. If a condom fails, therefore, and an individual becomes infected with HIV, there is potential for that person to accuse their partner of being 'reckless' for having withheld information that may have influenced their decision to have sex.

Assumed status and trust

Disclosing one's HIV status to an intimate partner can be extremely difficult. Many people have difficulty coming to terms with having HIV and remain in denial of their condition. The fear of rejection and stigma can also prevent people from being honest, particularly if they are worried about friends, colleagues or members of their family finding out. Likewise, asking about someone else's status can be hard because of the risk of offending them, or 'spoiling the moment'. In such circumstances, many people choose to make assumptions instead.

Ironically, this is particularly true in high-prevalence areas or among high-risk groups where virtually everyone has heard of HIV. A positive person who engages in casual sex with a negative person may, for example, assume that by failing to suggest the use of a condom or failing to ask about status, the negative partner is either already positive themselves or does not care about the risks of HIV. Likewise, a negative person may assume that by not using a condom and not talking about status, their partner must be negative too:

'If she was HIV+, she'd ask me to use a condom...' or 'He's not using a condom, so he must be HIV+, like me'.

There is also the issue of trust. Most would agree that a relationship can only work if both partners have faith in each other to be honest and truthful. But when one partner consistently lies or deceives the other, where does the blame lie? With the person who has been deceptive, or with the person who has been naive enough to trust them?

Police investigations

There have been cases in the UK and abroad, where police have assumed that because HIV transmission can now be a criminal offence, it is acceptable to fully investigate any HIV+ person about whom they receive a complaint. In some cases, this will involve actively raiding the accused's home for evidence of HIV+ status or demanding medical records from HIV clinics. Police have also been known to track down past partners to inform them of their risk, or even to persuade them to testify against the accused individual.

How such activities fit in to national laws about privacy and confidentiality needs to be assessed very carefully, and HIV-positive people need to be aware of their rights if ever they undergo such an investigation. It also needs to be made very clear who (the police or public health officers) should trace and contact previous partners, how this should be done to ensure proper counselling and help is provided. Questions about whether anyone has the right to trace and contact previous partners if the person concerned does not give consent for this to happen also need to be addressed.

Reasons for prosecuting

Sometimes a lack of knowledge regarding HIV-associated risk and what a prosecution may entail could lead to someone making a formal complaint before they later realise it is not in their interest to do so. An impulsive overreaction upon being diagnosed, due to a misunderstanding of transmission risk, or acting out of vengeance against a former partner following a bad break-up, for example, could lead someone in the heat of the moment to try and take legal action. Poor advice by solicitors or, as mentioned, police may encourage a complainant to believe they have a solid case when it is unlikely to lead to conviction. Furthermore, they may later doubt that the defendant was the source of their infection. Complainants may also be led to believe they are entitled to complete anonymity only to find their entire sexual history dragged publicly through the courts in a case that was unlikely to end in conviction anyway.

Criminal prosecution: right or wrong?

Given the ambiguities and difficulties outlined above, it is apparent that any form of legislation on the issue needs to be clear about what forms of transmission are and are not covered. There are generally three broad schools of thought on how this should work:

No criminalisation at all

A few people argue that criminal charges should never be brought for transmitting HIV, no matter what the circumstances. HIV is a virus that acts under its own rules of nature, they say, and therefore the laws of man should not apply. Banning any prosecution for HIV transmission would therefore make the whole issue a lot simpler. Many would consider this rule to pose a threat to public health by leaving individuals who wish to do harm immune to prosecution.

Criminalisation for intentional transmission only

Generally this is the sort of policy that most AIDS organisations, public health officials and civil rights groups favour. They argue that by restricting the law to cases of intentional rather than reckless transmission, it would greatly reduce the confusion amongst HIV+ people over what is legal and what is not. It would also cut down on the number of HIV+ people being criminalised unfairly, while allowing those who truly deserve prosecution to be brought to trial. In cases of reckless or accidental transmission, most agree that education and counselling is a more effective prevention method than imprisonment or fines.

Furthermore, it has been argued that even in cases of intentional transmission the wording of laws used to prosecute should not be HIV-specific. Instead, existing criminal law should be used so as not to further stigmatise people with HIV as a whole.

Criminalisation for all forms of transmission

Many states and countries now allow the prosecution of HIV-positive people for all forms of transmission, including reckless and accidental, and even for exposure where no transmission has taken place. Some have specific laws permitting this, others use more general criminal laws to obtain a conviction. As with any type of criminal trial, once one prosecution is successfully achieved, it sets a precedent for future trials, and makes lawyers more likely to take on similar cases. This growing trend is of particular concern for many organisations trying to advocate on behalf of HIV+ people around the world.

How does criminalisation affect the lives of HIV+ people?

While most HIV+ people practise very safe sex, and would never have cause to be taken to court, many say that the issue of criminalisation still affects them. A recent survey by researchers from the Sigma research team at Portsmouth University, for example, found that 90% of the HIV+ people they interviewed were critical of the growing trend for criminalisation of reckless HIV transmission. Most said this was because they believed that the responsibility for protected sex should be shared, or because they thought criminalisation increased the stigma they faced. A number also said they believed that criminalisation was a step back towards the culture of 'blame' that surrounded the early years of the epidemic.

Right or wrong, however, criminalisation does mean that there is now an extra concern for any HIV+ person who decides to have a sexual relationship, and many HIV organisations are finding that they have to take the issue into consideration when giving out advice. In its booklet *Should I tell?* about HIV disclosure, for example, the UK charity THT decided to change a number of pages to reflect the fact that emotional and sexual concerns are no longer the only issue that needs to be addressed in the bedroom – legal issues have to be taken into consideration too.

Updated 9 December 2008

⇨ The above information is an extract from the article 'Criminal transmission of HIV' and is reprinted with kind permission from AVERT. To view the full text of this article or to find out more about this and other related issues, please visit the AVERT website at www.avert.org

© AVERT

Diseased theories

Some conspiracy theories are easy enough to dismiss, but the ones about HIV can have a far more deadly effect

By Priya Shetty

You're in a bar in a vibrant city somewhere around the globe – Cape Town or Mumbai perhaps – having a drink with friends. You've been chatting to someone all night and think you might get lucky. You know that catching something like HIV is no laughing matter, so do you (a) make sure you have condoms before you go over to their place or (b) cross your legs and wait till you're married? If you live in Africa, the answer had better be (b), according to the head of the Catholic Church in Mozambique (and if you live in the West, and thought that people in India or Africa would default to (b) because of conservative cultural mores, well, get real).

Francisco Chimoio made headlines last week with his claim that European-made condoms are deliberately laced with the HIV virus. This sabotage, he says, was intended to wipe out 'the African people'. But these aren't just whacky comments that can be filed under 'strange things that religious extremists say'. The fact that Chimoio isn't the first, and certainly won't be the last, to spout HIV conspiracy theories points to the denial that several political and religious leaders are in about the mammoth challenges that developing countries face in trying to defeat the disease.

To halt the HIV epidemic, poor countries need to revamp their health systems, which means training more staff and building proper infrastructure. Not only that, unlike with malaria or TB – the other two in the trilogy of big diseases that hit poor nations hardest – defeating HIV requires enormous social change, both by empowering women and dealing with morally taboo issues like prostitution and drugs. Faced with the Herculean effort involved in doing what will really work, it is easier for religious and political leaders to shout moral messages from their pulpits and parliaments, and then claim western plots to kill Africans

when those messages don't have the desired effect.

Religious leaders have always been in a quandary with HIV – the disease is inextricably linked to sex and drugs, with sex workers, gay men and injecting drug users particularly at risk of infection. Rather than engage with the complexity of these issues, the Catholic Church's response has been to preach abstinence, a position taken up by the US government, which demands that much of the money it donates to HIV/AIDS programmes must be spent promoting abstinence. To make sure that Catholics aren't tempted to indulge in a spot of naughty but protected sex, the Vatican also declared that condoms had tiny holes that HIV could pass through. After all, it's not a real fight if you're not trashing the opposition.

Worryingly, some HIV conspiracy theorists are key political figures. Manto Tshabalala-Msimang, South Africa's health minister, earned herself the moniker 'Dr Beetroot' because of her promotion of garlic and beetroot as AIDS remedies – she believes that anti-HIV drugs are toxic. Clearly she is following the party line, because President Thabo Mbeki has famously denied that the HIV virus is the sole cause of AIDS.

Why does HIV draw out these bizarre statements? Perhaps because conspiracy theories tend to cluster around a social phenomenon where the reality is too hard to stomach – much-loved figures such as Elvis dying or JFK being shot, or the Earth slowly burning to a crisp as its climate changes. It wouldn't be hard to put the Rasputin-like HIV virus in this category, given that despite millions of dollars and years of effort, it continues to ravage the world and seems no closer to being snuffed out than when it first emerged in the 1980s.

Some conspiracy theories are easy to dismiss, but the ones about HIV are far more deadly. Abstinence and fidelity aren't practical ways of stopping the spread of HIV – the allure of sex is too strong for any society to pretend otherwise. The HIV epidemic continues to destroy many African countries – in southern Africa, about one in five people are infected. Conspiracy theories merely serve to divert attention from the fact that moral messages about HIV simply don't work.

South Africa has the second largest number of people with HIV in the entire world. People attend more funerals there than they do weddings. Faced with such colossal problems, its political leaders have taken to the equivalent of putting their fingers in their ears and humming to drown out the insistent message that they need to confront the epidemic head-on.

What will confronting it really mean? Well for one thing, when it comes to sex, only a grown up attitude is going to work – women need to feel they can use contraception (not only to protect themselves but to ensure they don't pass the virus on to their babies). Wresting sexual autonomy from men in cultures that still believe women are the weaker sex won't be easy. Whatever their rights or wrongs, drugs, prostitution, and sex outside marriage are a fact of life; pretending otherwise will do nothing to stop the AIDS epidemic, but education about the risks of HIV, if done in the right way, can achieve a lot.

It isn't that morality (religious or otherwise) shouldn't guide healthcare – arguably the human rights framework that demands healthcare for all is a type of morality in itself. But hiding behind certain types of morality and refusing to acknowledge that some moral judgements aren't worth making will actually do more harm than good.

1 October 2007

Record UK HIV diagnoses

New figures reveal growing number of heterosexuals acquiring HIV within the UK

The latest figures from the Health Protection Agency reveal that the number of people living with HIV in the UK increased to an estimated 77,400 in 2007, with 7,734 new diagnoses in 2007 alone. Although high, the number of people diagnosed with HIV each year seems to have reached a plateau – but this disguises more worrying trends.

Increase in heterosexual transmission in the UK

The estimated number of HIV-positive people diagnosed who were infected through heterosexual contact within the UK has increased from 540 new diagnoses in 2003 to 960 in 2007, and has doubled from 11 per cent to 23 per cent as a proportion of all het-erosexual diagnoses in this period.

Need to get better at diagnosing HIV early

Over a quarter (28 per cent) of people living with HIV are unaware of their infection and many of those that are diagnosed are being diagnosed late – after the point at which they should have started treatment. 42 per cent of heterosexual men and 36 per cent of heterosexual women were diagnosed late compared to 19 per cent of gay or bisexual men. People diagnosed

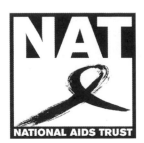

late are 13 times more likely to die within a year of diagnosis.

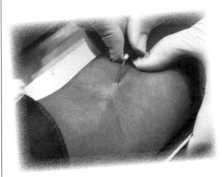

Many people risking health by delaying treatment

The statistics also highlight an area of growing concern – the number of people choosing not to start or to delay starting treatment. Almost one in five people with diagnosed HIV who are at the point when it is recommended treatment begin have nevertheless made the decision not to start treatment.

Deborah Jack, Chief Executive of NAT (National AIDS Trust), comments:

> **The number of people living with HIV in the UK increased to an estimated 77,400 in 2007, with 7,734 new diagnoses in 2007 alone**

'Each year a significant number of people are diagnosed with HIV, showing we still have much more to do to reduce ongoing HIV infection in the UK. Funding for prevention and testing must be increased and the Government must begin to take seriously the public health challenge of HIV in the UK, as it is growing each year.

'Most worrying is the number of people who should be on HIV treatment but who in fact are not – whether because they are unaware of their infection or because they are opting not to start treatment when recommended. Treatment for HIV has revolutionised the condition and people with HIV can now expect a good life expectancy if they are diagnosed early and take their medication as advised. By not getting treatment, people are risking their health.'

1 December 2008

⇨ The above information is reprinted with kind permission from the National AIDS Trust. Visit www.worldaidsday.org.uk for more information.

© National AIDS Trust

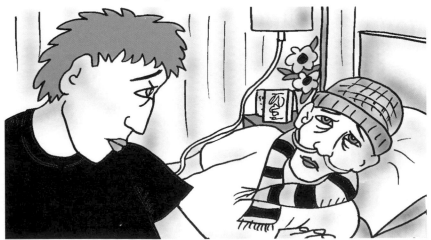

AIDS epidemic update

UK regional summary

Heterosexually acquired HIV infections, most of which were in immigrants and migrants, formed the largest proportion (42%) of new HIV infections diagnosed in Western Europe in 2006. A little under one-third (29%) of newly diagnosed HIV infections were attributable to unsafe sex between men, while a diminishing proportion of diagnoses (6%) were reported in injecting drug users (EuroHIV, 2007).

In Western and Central Europe, the United Kingdom continues to have a large HIV epidemic, together with France, Italy and Spain. The annual number of newly diagnosed HIV infections has more than doubled in the United Kingdom, from 4,152 in 2001 to 8,925 in 2006 (EuroHIV, 2007). The country also has one of the highest rates of new HIV diagnoses in Western and Central Europe: 149 per one million population in 2006, which is exceeded only by Portugal's 205 per one million population (EuroHIV, 2007).

The HIV epidemic continues to be concentrated in London, which accounted for 41% of new HIV diagnoses in 2006. However, significant increases in new diagnoses have occurred in the East Midlands, Northern Ireland and Wales (Health Protection Agency, 2007).

The continued increase in HIV diagnoses reported in the United Kingdom is due mainly to sustained levels of newly acquired infections in men who have sex with men, an increase in diagnoses among heterosexual men and women who acquired their infection in a high-prevalence country (mainly in sub-Saharan Africa and the Caribbean), and improved reporting due to increased and earlier HIV testing.

Men who have sex with men continue to be the population group most at risk of acquiring HIV within the United Kingdom. An estimated 82% of men who have sex with men diagnosed with HIV in 2006 probably acquired their infection in the United Kingdom (compared with 18% for heterosexual men and women) (Health Protection Agency, 2007). The number of new HIV diagnoses in men who have sex with men almost doubled between 2001 and 2006, from 1,434 to 2,597 (EuroHIV, 2007). However, it is unclear whether that increase reflects changing HIV incidence or changes in testing in this population group (Health Protection Agency, 2006; Dougan et al., 2007).

In other countries in this region, approximately one-third of persons (32% in 2005) newly diagnosed with HIV are unaware of their infection (Health Protection Agency, 2006). Even larger proportions of HIV-infected men who have sex with men remain unaware of their HIV status. For example, a five-city survey in bars, clubs and saunas frequented by homosexual men found that 41% of men who tested HIV-positive had been previously undiagnosed (Williamson et al., 2006).

The number of HIV diagnoses in people who acquired their infection through unprotected heterosexual intercourse almost doubled, from 2,379 in 2001 to 4,514 in 2006 (EuroHIV, 2006, 2007). Here, too, increased uptake of HIV testing among people attending genitourinary clinics (which reached 82% in 2005) might have been a factor in that rising trend. Most of the HIV diagnoses attributed to unprotected heterosexual intercourse were in persons who had been infected in a high-prevalence country, mainly in sub-Saharan Africa.

As in other countries in this region, there continues to be late HIV diagnosis among African and other ethnic minority adults. Approximately 40% of persons from those population groups who tested HIV-positive in 2005 were diagnosed late, and they were considerably more likely to die within a year of their HIV diagnosis (compared with persons whose infections were detected earlier)

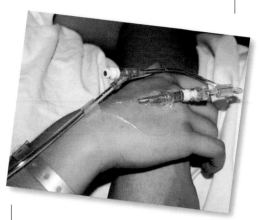

(Health Protection Agency, 2006). Research in the Midlands and southern England suggests that stigma and fear of discrimination discourage a large proportion of Africans in the United Kingdom from testing for HIV (Elam et al., 2006).

Infection as a result of exposure to contaminated drug injecting equipment accounts for a small number of HIV cases (131 new diagnoses in 2006) in the United Kingdom's HIV epidemic (Health Protection Agency, 2007). Nevertheless, HIV infections continue to be found among injecting drug users. Outside London, estimated prevalence among injecting drug users rose from 0.5% in 2003 to 1.2% in 2005 (Health Protection Agency, 2006).

Overall, data such as these suggest that there is scope for improvement in the United Kingdom's AIDS response. For example, coverage of HIV testing could be increased and focused, and appropriate prevention programmes could be expanded among population groups that are at highest risk of HIV infection.
March 2008

⇨ The above information is an extract from the document *North America, Western and Central Europe – AIDS epidemic update, regional summary* and is reprinted with kind permission from UNAIDS and the World Health Organisation. Visit www.who.int and www.unaids.org for more information.
© WHO/UNAIDS

Stigmatising HIV and AIDS

Complacency and stigma prevalent as cases of HIV in UK increase

New research published today indicates that 1 in 7 young people interviewed in Britain would not be willing to remain friends with someone if they had HIV and only 32% are worried about getting HIV. The international Ipsos MORI survey, commissioned by the British Red Cross, indicates a worrying level of complacency and stigma towards HIV in Britain today despite last week's report from UNAIDS, which found that HIV is on the rise in the UK.

The British Red Cross is releasing these research findings as it launches a major new campaign today (26 November) to raise awareness of the global issue of HIV. The campaign 'HIV: What's the story?', launched ahead of World AIDS Day, is aimed at teenagers and young adults and is delivered via digital media and social networking sites to ensure maximum exposure amongst its target audience.

The level of stigma in Britain is similar to results from South Africa, where almost a fifth of young people interviewed would not be willing to remain friends with someone with HIV. With more than 5 million people living with HIV, South Africa is the country with the largest number of HIV infections in the world. In Kyrgyzstan, where HIV is an emerging problem, almost half of young people interviewed said they would not remain friends with a person living with HIV. In Ethiopia, almost a quarter (23%) of those interviewed would not be willing to remain friends with someone with HIV.

Alyson Lewis, HIV Advisor at the British Red Cross, said: 'The stigma and secrecy attached to HIV is having a direct impact on young people's ability worldwide to access information and talk openly about their fears and concerns about the spread of this devastating pandemic.' She continued: 'Almost half of British young people interviewed would want to keep it a secret if a member of their family was living with HIV. Many young people view HIV as a shameful secret, and we need to ensure that we demystify these fears and help young people to be more aware of the risks and how to protect themselves.'

The British Red Cross supports peer education programmes at home and abroad, which enable young people to gain and share information and skills. There are thousands of young peer educators who volunteer for the Red Cross who are passionate in their ambition to help reduce stigma and discrimination towards HIV.

Nicola Waghorn (22), a Red Cross peer educator from Brighton, said: 'I don't think young people in the UK really know that much about HIV. Many of them don't know enough about the risks involved.' She continued: 'I can help my friends understand more by passing on information that I know and correcting their misunderstandings.'

'I know what HIV is doing to my society,' said Hamza (20), Red Cross peer educator in Ethiopia. 'I think that if I teach one person about HIV then they can go back and teach their family. In this way awareness will come.'

Lewis added: 'Our priority is to reduce stigma and promote human dignity for all people living with HIV. This campaign succeeds in that it enables young people from all over the world to talk about their experiences in their own words.'
26 November 2007

⇨ The above information is reprinted with kind permission from the British Red Cross. Visit www.redcross.org.uk/hiv for more information.
© British Red Cross

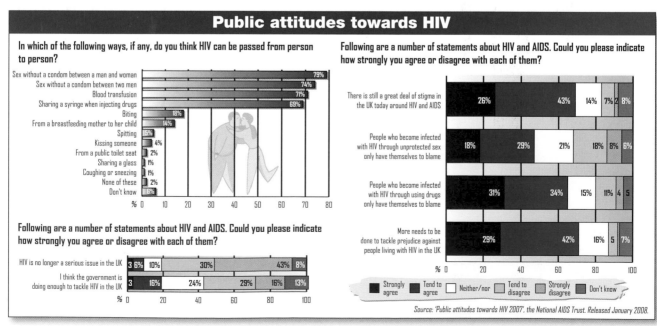

Public attitudes towards HIV

In which of the following ways, if any, do you think HIV can be passed from person to person?

- Sex without a condom between a man and woman — 79%
- Sex without a condom between two men — 74%
- Blood transfusion — 71%
- Sharing a syringe when injecting drugs — 69%
- Biting — 18%
- From a breastfeeding mother to her child — 14%
- Spitting — 5%
- Kissing someone — 4%
- From a public toilet seat — 2%
- Sharing a glass — 1%
- Coughing or sneezing — 1%
- None of these — 2%
- Don't know — 6%

Following are a number of statements about HIV and AIDS. Could you please indicate how strongly you agree or disagree with each of them?

- HIV is no longer a serious issue in the UK — 3% / 6% / 10% / 30% / 43% / 8%
- I think the government is doing enough to tackle HIV in the UK — 3% / 16% / 24% / 29% / 16% / 13%

Following are a number of statements about HIV and AIDS. Could you please indicate how strongly you agree or disagree with each of them?

- There is still a great deal of stigma in the UK today around HIV and AIDS — 26% / 43% / 14% / 7% / 2% / 8%
- People who become infected with HIV through unprotected sex only have themselves to blame — 18% / 29% / 21% / 18% / 8% / 6%
- People who become infected with HIV through using drugs only have themselves to blame — 31% / 34% / 15% / 11% / 4 / 5
- More needs to be done to tackle prejudice against people living with HIV in the UK — 29% / 42% / 16% / 5 / 7%

Legend: Strongly agree / Tend to agree / Neither/nor / Tend to disagree / Strongly disagree / Don't know

Source: 'Public attitudes towards HIV 2007', the National AIDS Trust. Released January 2008.

Step into the future

I'm not talking about wormholes, intergalactic travel or alien life. Instead, I am referring to time

Let me take you back to the 1970s…

In the music charts we had David Bowie, Elton John and some of the great disco classics on vinyl. Fashion saw never-to-be-forgotten platform shoes, mini-skirts and the flower-power peace-loving hippies. Over 35 years ago a DHSS Expert Group on the Treatment of Haemophilia recommended that the NHS should be self-sufficient in blood products as soon as possible. The huge risk of hepatitis in treatment was known.

Funds were assigned to this but they failed, miserably, to be used and thus began the destruction of the innocent lives of thousands due to maladministration and false promises, Britain did not become self-sufficient. Indeed, it is something that even to this day has still not been achieved.

Fast forward to the 1980s…

We had Band-Aid at number one with Do They Know It's Christmas? We listened to Madonna, Kylie and Sister Sledge on our cassette walkmans. The world's eyes focused on Ethiopia while power suits, yuppies and big hair were symbols of the era. One of the most memorable public figures was the then occupant of number 10 Downing Street, Margaret Thatcher. HIV/AIDS brought the world to its knees through fear and 1,200 haemophiliacs became infected while thousands more were also infected with what we now call hepatitis C. Terror was felt across the globe as our community was, along with others, so dramatically hit. We listened in total disbelief to the impact it was having as each day saw more and more deaths. We, the patients, were put through undignified procedures and questions, test after test, as we watched our friends and loved ones leave us for ever.

Skip into the 1990s…

Take That were the boy kings of pop with record CD sales. Erasure went all Abba-esque while Michael Jackson made us think about the planet with Earth Song. Rock idol Freddie Mercury took his final bow. In 1992 US Senator Mike Huckabee made this statement: 'steps should be taken that would isolate carriers of this plague…' He was referring to carriers of HIV; the virus that can lead to AIDS. He went on to say: 'It is the first time in civilisation in which the carriers of a genuine plague have not been isolated….' The country was now under the power of New Labour and Tony Blair's government would make even more promises and apparently learn more lessons. Meanwhile, as still more people died from multiple viruses, vCJD was being injected into the veins of haemophiliacs. The nation lost their Queen of Hearts but many lost much, much more.

Leap forward to 2007…

Beyoncé, Mika and the newly re-grouped Take That topped the music charts once again. Our new government and official bodies confidently told us that even more lessons have been learned and we have nothing to worry about. In fact, during his first speech as Prime Minister in June last year, Gordon Brown said:

> **HIV/AIDS brought the world to its knees through fear and 1200 haemophiliacs became infected while thousands more were also infected with what we now call Hepatitis C**

'I heard the need for change.' He told us that he '…will continue to listen and learn from the British people to deliver changes to the country'. He then added that his government would also change to build people's trust in the government and change to protect and extend the British way of life…

So here it is: Happy 2008…

As I sit here and write this article, January not only deeply concerns me but the shiver sent up my spine is one I have become all too familiar with: the gut-wrenching feeling that I get when I hear about our safety and lives, even

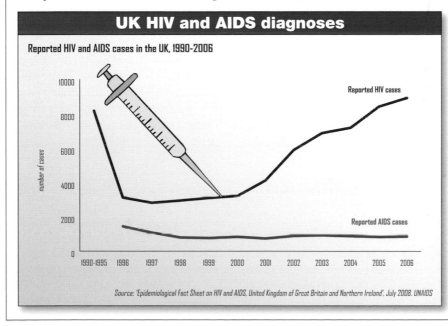

UK HIV and AIDS diagnoses

Reported HIV and AIDS cases in the UK, 1990-2006

Source: 'Epidemiological Fact Sheet on HIV and AIDS. United Kingdom of Great Britain and Northern Ireland'. July 2008. UNAIDS

after all these years, still being put on the line. The headlines and news from the first month of this year outline more betrayal and neglect:

⇨ January 1st, 2008: Britain's biggest blood processing lab is filthy and could pose a danger to patients, a leaked document reveals. Health inspectors blasted the Government-owned Bio Products Laboratory after exposing 90 'major failures'.

⇨ January 3rd, 2008: Japan PM apologises for Tainted Blood [a scandal in the 1980s in which over 1,000 Japanese haemophiliacs contracted HIV through contaminated blood products].

⇨ January 10th, 2008: 18 British soldiers wounded in action are facing HIV fears after it emerged they may have been given US front-line contaminated blood.

⇨ January 11th, 2008: Shanghai parents to sue for tainted blood.

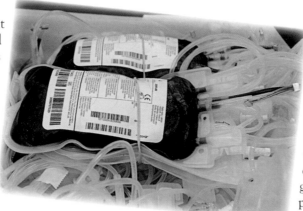

It has been known for individuals to contract the HIV virus through contaminated blood transfusions

⇨ January 12th, 2008: 31 Australian troops wounded in Afghanistan are urgently being checked to see whether they have been exposed to contaminated blood.

⇨ January 26th, 2008: The NHS has owned up to seven new breaches of security involving patient details. Health secretary faces questions over campaign donations. A statement published from Alan Johnson's campaign office said...

'So to be clear, there was never any wrongdoing', a sentence used far too conveniently over the years with the notion that it makes everything all right.

These do not inspire confidence, do they? I feel obliged to ask, is this care or selective culling? Finally at the time this goes to print, Lord Archer's public inquiry team [into NHS supply of contaminated blood] have been silent since 19 September 2007 with no formal statement or reason. The trust we gave them and the hope they gave us in moving closer to justice has gradually dwindled. Here we are again left wondering what will become of us. *By Mark Ward of the Tainted Blood team. www.taintedblood.info*

⇨ Information from Positive Nation. Visit www.positivenation.co.uk for more information.

© Sugar media

Getting tested for HIV

Information from Staying Alive

Although it can be a frightening prospect, knowing your HIV status (whether you are HIV-positive or HIV-negative) can help you make important decisions and plans for the future. There are many reasons why you might consider getting tested. Here are some of the main reasons you may want talk with a health care provider about taking a test:

⇨ had sexual intercourse (vaginal, oral, or anal) without a condom or dental dam (thin, square pieces of latex or polyurethane for oral sex)

⇨ learned that a partner was not monogamous (had sex with another partner)

⇨ have been sexually assaulted

⇨ had a condom break during sex

⇨ shared needles or syringes, or found out that a partner has shared needles

⇨ had multiple sexual partners

⇨ discovered that a partner has been exposed to HIV or learned that

a past or current partner is HIV-positive

⇨ had a recent diagnosis of another sexually transmitted infection (STI)

⇨ are pregnant.

How the test works

When you get an HIV test, a lab tests your blood for antibodies that your immune system produces to fight off the HIV virus. Although these antibodies can't destroy the virus, their presence in the blood can be used to confirm that you've been infected. If the test detects antibodies then you are HIV-positive.

When to get tested

Most blood tests can detect HIV infection within three months of initial exposure to the virus, but it can sometimes take up to six months for antibodies to reach detectable levels. It is generally recommended that you take a test six months after

the last possible exposure. If you get tested shortly after exposure then you should take another test a few months later to confirm the result.

What to do next

Getting the results of your HIV test is an emotional event and whatever the outcome, you need to think about what to do next.

If you are HIV-negative, make sure that you continue to protect yourself at all times. If you are having sex, ensure that you're using condoms correctly and that you use one every time. If you inject drugs, be sure to use sterilised needles and syringes each time, and don't share your equipment. You should also take another test about six months later to confirm the negative result.

If you are HIV-positive, the sooner you take steps to protect your health, the better. Medical treatment and a healthy lifestyle can help you stay well. The proper treatment may delay the onset of AIDS and prevent some life-threatening conditions. You should...

⇨ See a doctor, even if you don't feel sick. If possible, see a doctor who has experience treating HIV. Consulting someone about your treatment options is an important first step.

⇨ Get a tuberculosis test done. TB often goes hand-in-hand with HIV – you may already be infected with TB and not know it. TB is a serious illness but can be treated successfully if caught early.

⇨ Be good to your immune system. Smoking cigarettes, drinking too much alcohol or using other recreational drugs can weaken your immune system. If you need help quitting, talk to your doctor about substance abuse programmes.

⇨ Find a support system. The emotional and physical challenges ahead can be difficult and having people around who understand what you're going through can be an enormous help. Ask your doctor about counsellors and support groups.

⇨ The above information is reprinted with kind permission from Staying Alive. Visit www.staying-alive.org for more information.

© Staying Alive

Living with HIV

Information from the Terrence Higgins Trust

My name's Alison and I am a 28-year-old heterosexual living near the south coast in England. I am pretty sure I became infected with HIV after a very unpleasant gap-year experience in Africa when I was 19.

On my return home, my GP arranged my HIV test and made sure that a local health advisor was available when I got my results, to give my mother and me support. This was all handled really sensitively, but was an incredibly stressful and traumatic experience in itself.

Since then my health has been fine and I am monitored by my local genito-urinary medicine (GUM) clinic a couple of times a year. I am lucky that I still haven't needed to go onto medication and I really hope this situation lasts as long as possible.

Personal feelings
I have told my closest friends and family and they have been great, but they don't really know what it is like to live with HIV. Over time I have managed to think about it less and less as this helps me not to worry and lets me get on with my life. But from time to time I get really scared about getting really ill – I guess I am a bit paranoid – and I do sink into a bit of a gloomy mood about it all.

Discrimination
I haven't experienced discrimination, but that is because I haven't been very open about my status. I really fear discrimination and prejudice and this stops me from being open with most people and probably adds to the isolation I feel. I feel stuck with my job as I know that they have an HIV non-disclosure and non-discrimination policy and a good pension. I don't know what I would face in another job.

Relationships
I only know one other person living with HIV, who is someone I met through the GUM clinic I was monitored at while I was at university. It made such a big difference meeting someone else who knew what I was going through.

The hardest thing was telling subsequent boyfriends. If you don't tell, you aren't having an honest relationship, so how can you really go anywhere with it? If you do tell and it's early days and doesn't work out, that is someone out there you can't really trust who knows something about you, which they could then use to ruin your life. It would make me feel so vulnerable.

I was so incredibly lucky to meet my now husband. I told him straight away. It was a gamble, but it meant that we were honest with each other from the start. He has been great and even got some information leaflets from THT to learn more about HIV. It makes me so sad that I will never be able to have unprotected sex with him.

⇨ The above information is reprinted with kind permission from the Terrence Higgins Trust. Visit www.tht.org.uk for more information.

© Terrence Higgins Trust

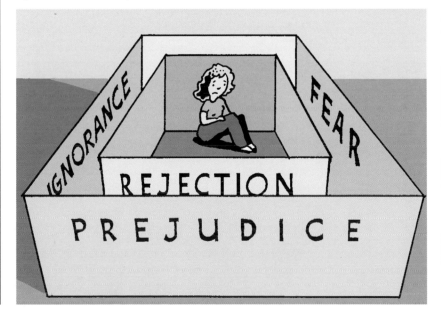

HIV and gay men

HPA warns of continuing HIV and STI epidemic in gay men

An estimated 73,000 adults are now living with HIV in the UK, according to the Health Protection Agency's latest report on the UK's sexual health. This figure includes both those who have been diagnosed and also around a third (21,600) who remain unaware of their HIV status.

Dr Valerie Delpech, Head of HIV surveillance at the Agency, said, 'Figures received so far for 2006, show 7,093 people were diagnosed with HIV in the UK. We expect this number to rise to an estimated 7,800 when all reports are received, a comparable figure to the 7,900 received in 2005.'

Dr Delpech went on to say, 'We are still seeing high levels of HIV transmission in gay men in whom we anticipate that there will have been just over 2,700 new diagnoses of HIV infection in 2006. In recent years we have seen steady increases in all sexually transmitted infections (STI), including HIV, in gay men and since 2003, the number of HIV diagnoses reported annually has consistently increased and exceeded the annual number of diagnoses throughout the 1980s and 1990s.'

Increased testing will have contributed in part to these recent high numbers of HIV diagnoses, but there is no suggestion that the overall level of underlying HIV transmission in gay men has fallen. Unprotected sex continues to be a very high risk activity for HIV and STI transmission in this group.

'Sexual health of young adults has worsened in 2006 with increases in sexually transmitted herpes and warts viruses. One in ten young adults screened through the National Chlamydia Screening Programme in 2006 tested positive for the infection,' said Dr Delpech.

In 2006, there were an estimated 750 new HIV diagnoses thought to be due to heterosexual HIV transmission within the UK, many in black ethnic minority communities. This compares to an estimated 700 cases reported in 2005 and 500 in 2003, showing that heterosexual HIV transmission is steadily increasing.

The number of cases who may have acquired HIV heterosexually in Africa has remained stable. When all reports are received this number will be around 3,450 in 2006 compared to 3,700 the previous year and a peak of 3,850 in 2003.

Professor Pete Borriello, Director of the HPA's Centre for Infections, said: 'Our report, *Testing Times*, launched ahead of World AIDS Day allows us to review the sexual health of the nation and examine progress on preventing HIV and sexually transmitted infections in the UK.

'While there have been some encouraging developments in HIV and STI prevention in the last year, such as the increase in HIV testing, a marked reduction in waiting times at STI clinics and wider chlamydia testing for young adults, the total number of STI diagnoses increased 2.4% from 606,600 in 2005 to 621,300 in 2006.

'The control of HIV and STI transmission is a major public health challenge and testing for STIs, including HIV, in the UK needs to be increased still further. We recommend that gay men should have regular HIV tests, STI clinic attendees should be tested for HIV at every visit and young sexually active adults should be screened for chlamydia annually and after a partner change.

'We need to reinforce the safe sex message for gay men, young adults and the broader community. The best way to protect yourself from contracting an STI, including HIV, is by practising safer sex by using a condom with all new and casual partners. Any person who believes they may be at risk or has symptoms suggestive of a sexually transmitted infection should consult their doctor or attend a clinic. The sooner HIV and other STIs are diagnosed and treated, the less likely it is they will be passed on.'

Note

Testing Times is a report on HIV and STIs in the UK and is published by the Health Protection Agency and collaborators in time for World AIDS Day.
23 November 2007

⇨ The above information is reprinted with kind permission from the Health Protection Agency. Visit www.hpa.org.uk for more information. To read the HPA's *Sexually Transmitted Infections and Young People in the United Kingdom: 2008* report, please visit www. hpa.org.uk/web/HPAwebFile/ HPAweb_C/1215589015362
© *Health Protection Agency*

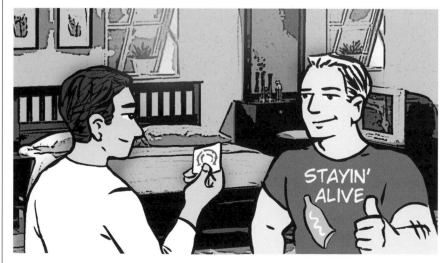

HIV prevention in the UK

Information from AVERT

Much of the early response to AIDS in the UK was driven by a fear that the epidemic would eventually spread beyond the minority groups it was originally associated with, and would have a major impact on the general population. In recent years, with HIV not spreading as widely as many had once predicted, HIV prevention efforts in the UK have been focused on the communities most affected, including gay men, people of African ethnicity and injecting drug users.

This shift in focus seems to have been accompanied by a decline in spending. Funding for HIV prevention in England and Wales is no longer 'ring-fenced', meaning it can be spent at the discretion of local health authorities; reports suggest that this has resulted in prevention money being spent on other areas of the health service. In Scotland, HIV prevention money is still ring-fenced by the Scottish Executive.

As levels of HIV in the UK are still rising, many AIDS organisations believe that national HIV prevention programmes should be reintroduced. These programmes should not only aim to reduce the transmission of the virus but also encourage uptake of HIV testing so that people know their status and, if infected, can access treatment.

HIV prevention amongst the general population

During the early years of the UK AIDS epidemic the government launched a variety of prevention campaigns imploring the British public not to 'die of ignorance'. The campaign used a variety of media to educate and inform people about how to protect themselves from HIV/AIDS.

The comprehensive anti-AIDS campaign in the 1980s was credited with raising awareness of how HIV is transmitted, encouraging condom use, and lowering rates of casual sex. It is thought that behaviour change prompted by this campaign may have prevented some HIV infections, although this has not been conclusively proven.

> **Educating people about the virus can help them to protect themselves and others, and can reduce the fear and stigma surrounding AIDS**

However, as time has passed and fears of a generalised epidemic in the UK have abated, there have been no further national HIV prevention campaigns aimed at the population as a whole. This means that a generation of sexually active young people have grown up largely complacent and unaware about the risks of becoming infected with HIV.

HIV education as prevention

HIV education is a vital component of HIV prevention strategies. Educating people about the virus can help them to protect themselves and others, and can reduce the fear and stigma surrounding AIDS.

A 2008 UK survey of people's attitudes to and knowledge of HIV conducted by the National AIDS Trust has found 'serious gaps' in people's knowledge about the virus. The study found that levels of understanding about HIV transmission in the UK have fallen significantly since the year 2000. It was found that in 2007, over 90 per cent of the British public did not fully understand the ways that HIV is transmitted, with Scotland and London reportedly being the least knowledgeable regions.

Deborah Jack, Chief Executive of the National AIDS Trust, emphasises the need to educate the general UK public about HIV:

Deaths of HIV-infected individuals

Deaths in HIV-infected individuals by year of death

Source: 'New HIV Diagnoses Surveillance Tables: UK data to the end of December 2007', December 2007. Health Protection Agency.

'Ignorance about HIV increases vulnerability to infection and also contributes to stigma and discrimination. The Government must reinvest in educating the public about HIV.'

HIV education in schools is one way to target young people with HIV prevention. In England and Wales, the government encourages secondary schools to teach pupils about HIV/AIDS as part of Sex and Relationships Education (SRE), although this is not a statutory subject on the National Curriculum. OFSTED – an official body that regulates schools in England – reported in 2007 that:

'Schools gave insufficient emphasis to teaching about HIV/AIDS. Despite the fact that it remains a significant health problem, pupils appear to be less concerned about HIV/AIDS than in the past.'

In Northern Ireland and Scotland, HIV/AIDS is not a compulsory part of school education either.

The Terrence Higgins Trust, amongst other organisations, believes that sex and relationships education should be a core part of the National Curriculum in the UK:

'The lack of good sex education means many young people are leaving school ignorant about HIV and safer sex. HIV is now the fastest growing serious health condition in the UK, and there is no cure. It's time to get our facts straight' (Nick Partridge, Chief Executive THT).

Men who have sex with men

Since the beginning of the UK AIDS epidemic, men who have sex with men (MSM) have been the group most at risk of HIV infection. It is thought that multiple prevention campaigns targeting the gay community may have had some positive effect on sexual behaviour and HIV incidence in the 1980s to mid-1990s. However, the number of new diagnoses in gay men in the UK has risen by 63% since 1997. While the increase may in part reflect a greater number of gay men coming forward for HIV testing, it is also feared that there has been a rise in unsafe sex due to complacency and the knowledge that HIV treatment is now available.

Gay men are currently the focus of a number of HIV prevention campaigns in the UK. An important nationally coordinated campaign is CHAPS, which is funded by the Department of Health and run by a partnership of organisations, led by the Terrence Higgins Trust. Its work is currently guided by a document called 'Making it Count', which sets out plans to reduce the number of HIV infections occurring through sex between men.

Another important campaign is the London Gay Men's HIV Prevention Partnership (LGMHPP) – a programme funded by several local health authorities across London, and run by seven AIDS-related organisations. Interventions carried out by the LGMHPP have included condom distribution at gay bars and clubs, adverts in the gay press, a volunteer-run helpline, and internet resources.

Despite campaigns to raise HIV awareness, there is evidence to suggest that many gay men are still ignoring safer sex messages. A study released in 2007 found that 18% of HIV-negative gay men had engaged in sex without using a condom. Worryingly, this figure rose to 37% for gay men who were HIV-positive.

HIV testing is an important part of preventing onward transmission of the virus. Although the number of MSM accessing HIV testing in GUM clinics has risen by 42% since 2003, the fact that 31% of gay men were unaware of their infection in 2006 indicates that there is a need for further promotion of HIV testing. Professor Peter Borriello, Director of the Health Protection Agency's Centre for Infections, says:

'Earlier diagnoses of HIV infection will give men access to treatment, improve their survival and reduce the risk of transmission to partners. I urge all gay men to test for HIV regularly.'

African communities in the UK

The Department of Health-funded National African HIV Prevention Programme (NAHIP) coordinates

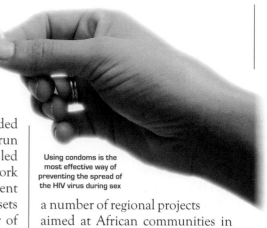

Using condoms is the most effective way of preventing the spread of the HIV virus during sex

a number of regional projects aimed at African communities in Britain. In May 2007 it launched the campaign 'beyond condoms', which aims to encourage condom use and greater openness about sexual health in the African community through outreach work, posters, leaflets and community workshops. A number of AIDS organisations working with African communities in the UK, including the African HIV Prevention Network (AHPN), are campaigning for more funding for HIV prevention activities amongst African communities.

It is important that any prevention work targeting African communities in the UK be supported by parallel activities that aim to reduce the problem of HIV-associated stigma and discrimination. A 2006 study found that fear of discrimination is stopping some people of African origin from accessing HIV testing services for fear of community reaction if their result were to be positive. Encouraging HIV testing uptake is a key part of preventing onward transmission of HIV in black communities. If people know their status they are less likely to pass the virus to others.

The Health Protection Agency (HPA) is concerned about the high proportion of black Africans in the UK who leave sexual health services unaware of their HIV status. It has been proposed that this problem could be overcome by testing high-risk groups for HIV under an opt-out policy, which means that they will automatically be tested for HIV unless they specifically ask not to be.

As the majority of Africans living with HIV in the UK were infected in sub-Saharan Africa, international aid from the British government for prevention programmes in developing countries can be seen as a strategy to reduce the number of people entering the UK who are already infected with the virus.

Injecting drug users

It is estimated that 131 injecting drug users (IDUs) became infected with HIV during 2006 – a fairly low number compared with some other countries. However, the proportion of IDUs living with HIV has increased, with an estimated one in fifty infected in 2006. This is around twice the level seen at the beginning of the decade.

The government funds some harm-reduction measures for injecting drug users, including needle exchange schemes and methadone substitution programmes. Needle exchange schemes are run by community pharmacies, the NHS and specialist providers to provide clean syringes to drug users to stop them sharing injecting equipment and transmitting HIV and other blood-borne viruses to others. In 2006, 90% of IDUs surveyed at specialist drug services in England reported that they had ever accessed a needle exchange service. Needle exchanges also provide information and support that can help people to stop taking drugs.

Doctors in the UK are permitted to prescribe methadone as a substitute for injected heroin. Through methadone substitution, users can also be helped to end their dependency on drugs.

Overall, the proportion of injecting drug users (IDUs) reporting that they had ever had a test for HIV increased from 50% in 1997 to 69% in 2006. Although this is a positive trend, in 2006 more than a third of HIV-infected IDUs who took part in an unlinked anonymous survey were not aware of their infection. This proportion is likely to be higher among IDUs who are not in contact with drug services.

Haemophiliacs and HIV transmission through blood products

In the late 1970s and early 1980s approximately 1,200 haemophiliacs were infected with HIV after being given imported plasma products. Three-quarters of the people infected in this way have since died.

In April 2007 an independent public inquiry began to investigate why the use of imported blood products continued after it emerged that the UK health department had been aware of the risk of HIV-contaminated blood as early as 1983. The UK was alerted to the threat of HIV-contaminated blood products imported from the USA, but believed that the benefits of the treatment for haemophiliacs outweighed the risks of HIV infection.

In 1985 the National Blood Service (NBS) introduced HIV screening for donated blood, and since this time only three people have been infected with HIV in this way.

Preventing mother-to-child transmission (PMTCT)

All pregnant women in the UK are routinely offered (and advised to take) an HIV test as part of their antenatal care. It's currently estimated that around 95% of HIV-infected women in the UK are diagnosed before delivery. Where it is established that a pregnant woman is HIV-positive, measures are taken to significantly reduce the chances of mother-to-child HIV transmission (MTCT), including the use of antiretroviral drugs.

These preventative measures have helped to keep the number of cases of MTCT occurring in the UK very low. Only 1.2% of all HIV-positive women who gave birth between 2000 and 2006 passed their HIV infection to their child. The majority of cases in which transmission of HIV did occur were due to either: late diagnosis of the mother (meaning that she did not start drug therapy at the recommended stage of pregnancy), poor drug adherence during pregnancy, or because of complications during birth.

Conclusion

In 2006, an estimated 7,800 persons were newly diagnosed with HIV in the UK. In order to stop this number rising further, preventing new HIV infections in the UK must be made a priority.

The British government needs to invest in HIV prevention, both for the general population and high prevalence groups, making sure that the earmarked money reaches its intended destination and is well managed and distributed. If this does not happen, knowledge about how HIV/AIDS is transmitted will continue to fall and the number of new HIV infections in the UK will rise.

⇨ The above information is reprinted with kind permission from AVERT. Visit www.avert.org for more information.

© AVERT

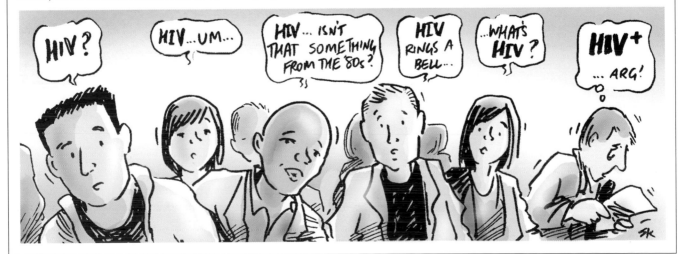

Condom use

Half the British public don't use condoms with new partners

Forty-nine per cent of the British public don't always use a condom when with a new sexual partner, according to the Ipsos MORI survey conducted for the National AIDS Trust (NAT). In National Condom Week NAT called for a new culture of condom use in the UK.

Where condoms are used by people who have had a new sexual partner within the last two years, the survey asked: 'When with a new sexual partner, at what point, if at all, would you stop using condoms?'

⇨ 24% of people who had a new sexual partner within the last two years said they would only stop using a condom once they and their partner had both been tested for HIV and other STIs, the one guaranteed way of knowing the state of your and your partner's sexual health.

⇨ a further 17% said they would always use a condom.

⇨ 53% of people who had had a new sexual partner within the last two years have put themselves at risk of an STI (sexually transmitted infection) when they stopped using condoms in a relationship.

The survey also revealed gaps in knowledge of the importance of condoms in preventing HIV transmission during sex. One in five (21%) failed to identify that HIV can be transmitted between a man and a woman who don't use a condom and over a quarter (26%) failed to identify that HIV can be transmitted between two men who don't use a condom.

The National AIDS Trust is calling on the Government to introduce:

⇨ condom use as an essential part of comprehensive, compulsory sex and relationships education in all schools.

⇨ condom advertising on TV and radio before the 9 o'clock watershed.

Deborah Jack, Chief Executive of the National AIDS Trust, said: 'The message is simple. Use condoms. And enjoy your safer sex life.'

August 2008

⇨ The above information is taken from Issue 13 of *SHINE* (Sexual Health Information News Exchange) and is reprinted with kind permission from NHS Sheffield. Visit www. sexualhealthsheffield.nhs.uk for more information.

© *Crown copyright*

Stop HIV: beyond ABC

Information from the Global AIDS Alliance

Did you know?

With over 33 million people infected with HIV worldwide and over 7,400 new infections every day, universal access to comprehensive HIV prevention services is essential. In 2007, roughly three million people became newly infected with HIV, including 470,000 children under the age of 15, most of whom were infected through mother-to-child transmission of the virus. HIV prevention does not have to be complicated in order to have a real impact on the spread of HIV/AIDS. But it does have to address the various needs of all populations at risk – from injection drug users to adult married women.

Understanding HIV infection and prevention

HIV can only be transmitted in a few ways: through sex, blood and mother-to-child transmission. Educating people about HIV and about the behaviours that put them at risk – such as unprotected sex and injection drug use – and enabling them to adopt safer behaviours are at the core of HIV prevention. Yet, preventing HIV requires a thorough understanding of the complex social, cultural, and economic factors that make some people more vulnerable to HIV infection than others. Worldwide, HIV is a disease of poverty and gender

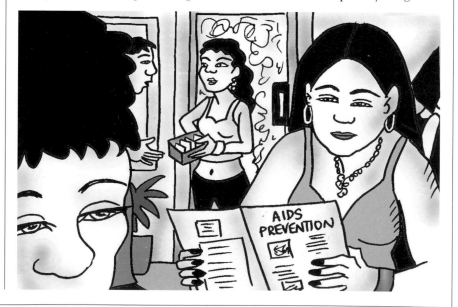

inequality. HIV prevalence statistics prove this: the highest rates of HIV occur in the poorest countries, where more women than men are infected, and young women are most at risk of acquiring HIV.

Lack of access to basic prevention services

According to UNAIDS, less than 20% of people at risk of HIV infection have access to basic prevention. In countries with a generalised epidemic (meaning that the virus is not restricted to a particular population, such as sex workers or injection drug users), everyone is at risk. In addition, only 11% of the world's pregnant women have access to services to prevent mother-to-child transmission (PMTCT), despite the fact that this is one of the cheapest and easiest prevention interventions available. Scaling up available prevention strategies in 125 low- and middle-income countries would prevent over 28 million new HIV infections between now and 2015 – the target date for achieving the Millennium Development Goals.

Stopping sexual transmission of HIV

HIV prevention includes a wide range of programmes and interventions that have been scientifically proven effective. One common approach to HIV prevention – the one endorsed by the US government through the President's Emergency Plan for AIDS Relief (PEPFAR) – is the 'ABC' model. ABC – abstinence, be faithful, use a condom – is potentially quite effective at preventing the spread of HIV. But it is essential that all three components be undertaken in a balanced and culturally-appropriate manner. For ABC to work, programmes that promote abstinence and fidelity must work together to delay sexual debut – the first time someone has sex – and limit the number of sexual partners. At the same time, condom education programs teach adolescents and adults about safer sex practices and provide them with access to male and female condoms (and hopefully someday to microbicides, too). The reality is that most people become sexually active in their late teens, young girls

in the global South are often forced into early marriages, and extramarital affairs are not uncommon. This means that everyone needs complete and accurate information about how to protect themselves against HIV when they do have sex, whether high-risk or not.

In addition to comprehensive HIV and condom education, people need to understand their sexual and reproductive health (SRH), including sexually transmitted infections, which increase the risk of acquiring HIV. One very important SRH service is prevention of mother-to-child HIV transmission, a highly cost-effective and successful intervention that must be made accessible to all pregnant women. Another element of SRH, male circumcision, has proven effective at protecting men from HIV, and should be carefully offered along with SRH and HIV counselling in a culturally appropriate setting. Violence against women and violence against children (VAW/C) is another important driver of the HIV pandemic. Sexuality and violence education programmes can help people negotiate safer, consensual sex, which can dramatically reduce the risks of HIV transmission. In addition, harm reduction is a fundamental HIV prevention approach for commercial sex workers and those engaged in transactional sex – often called poverty-driven sex or survival sex, because it involves people trading sex for things they need, like school fees, food, medicine, or money. For this vulnerable population, harm reduction includes education about HIV/AIDS and related risk factors, provision of condoms, and economic empowerment programmes.

Poverty and HIV/AIDS prevention

Because AIDS is a disease of poverty and because women are almost 70% of the world's poor, economic empowerment efforts are an important element of HIV prevention. Foremost among these is universal access to a free basic education. Primary education can reduce the impact of poverty, particularly on girls and women, decrease early marriage, facilitate family planning,

and increase gender equity and awareness of human rights – all of which can slow the spread of HIV. Programmes like microfinance schemes can have a direct impact on economic independence for those past schooling age, with benefits that are passed on to younger generations.

Stopping intravenous transmission of HIV

Although unprotected sex remains the primary cause of HIV transmission worldwide, blood and injection safety – both in health care settings and among drug users – is also a critical component of HIV prevention. Hundreds of thousands of HIV infections are caused each year through unsafe injections in health care settings; for example, through accidental needle pricks during vaccinations. Laboratory safety and access to clean syringes in health care settings are essential to prevent this method of HIV transmission. But harm reduction with injection drug users (IDUs) is also key, and often overlooked. Nearly one-third of all HIV infections outside Africa are attributed to injection drug use, yet only 5% of IDUs worldwide receive any HIV prevention services. Injection drug use is a particularly important factor in the HIV/AIDS epidemics of extremely populous, so-called 'second wave' countries like Russia and China, and in Vietnam, the newest PEPFAR focus country. Clean needle exchange and programmes to help people who wish to stop using injection drugs are best practices endorsed by the World Health Organisation and should be made widely available.

Prevention technologies

Finally, as HIV and AIDS continue to spread, decimating entire communities, it is urgent that increased resources be invested into new and underutilised technologies to prevent HIV. Female condoms should be made available at low cost around the world. Research into microbicides, which would allow women to protect themselves against HIV without their partner's knowledge or cooperation, and into a vaccine for HIV should receive greater investment from the global community.

What needs to be done?

In order to meet the Millennium Development Goals by 2015, much greater attention will need to be paid to the AIDS pandemic. As a result, United Nations member states have committed to achieving specific targets for universal access to HIV/AIDS services by 2010. The prevention targets include reducing AIDS cases by 25%, reducing the number of HIV-infected children by 50%, and increasing to 95% the proportion of young people who both correctly identify ways to prevent HIV and reject major misconceptions about HIV. These commitments must be kept if we are to slow and ultimately reverse the spread of HIV/AIDS.

Governments and multilateral agencies need to support comprehensive and fully funded HIV prevention programmes that do not impose ideological beliefs and that reflect the realities of people's lives. First and foremost, this means that ABC programmes must be conducted in a balanced manner, according to scientific evidence of what works and what doesn't. US law currently requires that one-third of all money spent on HIV prevention overseas supports abstinence-until-marriage programmes. Yet, a number of experts have reported that this requirement contradicts scientific evidence and is actually undermining efforts to stop the spread of HIV. For more information, take a look at reports on PEPFAR from the Government Accountability Office and the Institute of Medicine, both of which recommend that PEPFAR promote a comprehensive approach to HIV prevention.

Thankfully, the Global Fund to Fight AIDS, Tuberculosis and Malaria is providing much-needed balance to PEPFAR's emphasis on abstinence in poor, AIDS-affected countries. The Global Fund supports comprehensive ABC programming, as well as harm reduction for sex workers and IDUs, anti-violence programmes, comprehensive sexual and reproductive health services, health system strengthening, and other important components of HIV prevention. But the Global Fund must be fully funded, with the US and other wealthy donors increasing their contributions each year to help the Fund continue its current work and scale up programmes that have proven effective.

All HIV/AIDS programmes must adopt a model similar to the Global Fund's – one that integrates the diverse factors driving the spread of HIV. Many such programmes exist, and they need to be scaled up through national-level programmes so that everyone can benefit. Promising efforts include integration of HIV/AIDS and SRH services and social marketing for condoms. At the same time, stronger health systems are needed to ensure universal access to comprehensive HIV prevention services. This means more trained health care workers and adequate supplies and equipment, including condoms and HIV tests. Finally, mass media campaigns, such as Soul City in South Africa, that spread HIV awareness and prevention messages and combine SRH and VAW/C information with stigma reduction and promotion of safer sex, must reach all members of the population.

What is the Global AIDS Alliance doing?

The Global AIDS Alliance is committed to holding governments and stakeholders accountable for meeting their commitments, expressed in the Millennium Development Goals and HIV/AIDS universal access targets. GAA is simultaneously working to increase US support of the Global Fund and to hold PEPFAR accountable for implementing comprehensive, evidence-based programmes. We are also working with Congress to remove restrictions on programmes that can help prevent the spread of HIV among vulnerable groups. For example, GAA opposes the so-called prostitution pledge, which limits how US-funded AIDS groups can work with sex workers; the 'global gag rule' (also called the Mexico City Policy), which restricts US funding for groups that support or provide abortions; and the ban on clean needle exchange for IDUs. Other legislative efforts include increasing support for African health care workers and increasing US commitment to programmes that fight violence against women and violence against children through our Zero Tolerance campaign.

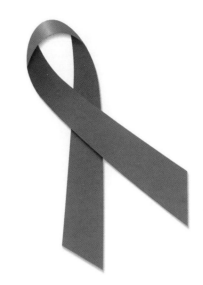

In addition, GAA views universal basic education as central to the HIV prevention agenda. We support Congressional efforts to increase funding for global education, work with the Education for All – Fast Track Initiative to increase its funding base and ensure that its programmes are of the highest possible quality, and advocate for global abolition of school fees with a range of international partners. GAA's prevention work also overlaps with our efforts to support orphans and other vulnerable children (OVC), who often lack access to education, are at particular risk of violence, and frequently resort to transactional sex for survival.

HIV prevention is complex, because each individual's vulnerability to HIV depends upon so many different social, cultural and economic factors. But there are many examples of holistic, multisectoral programmes that are having a positive impact, and GAA is committed to ensuring that these programmes are scaled up and fully funded so that the next generation does not face the risks of generalised HIV/AIDS epidemics.

⇨ The above information is reprinted with kind permission from the Global AIDS Alliance. Visit www.globalaidsalliance.org for more information.

© Global AIDS Alliance

3 million now receiving life-saving HIV drugs

But access to prevention and treatment still lacking for millions

The close of 2007 marks an important step in the history of the HIV/AIDS epidemic. Nearly 3 million people are now receiving antiretroviral therapy (ART) in low- and middle-income countries, according to a new report jointly launched today by WHO, UNAIDS and UNICEF.

Nearly 3 million people are now receiving anti-retroviral therapy (ART) in low- and middle-income countries

---

The report, *Towards universal access: scaling up priority HIV/AIDS interventions in the health sector*, also points to other gains. These include improved access to interventions aimed at preventing mother-to-child transmission of HIV (PMTCT), expanded testing and counselling, and greater country commitment to male circumcision in heavily affected regions of sub-Saharan Africa.

'This represents a remarkable achievement for public health,' said WHO Director-General Dr Margaret Chan. 'This proves that, with commitment and determination, all obstacles can be overcome. People living in resource-constrained settings can indeed be brought back to economically and socially productive lives by these drugs.'

Millions now accessing treatment

According to the authors of the report, the close of 2007 saw nearly 1 million more people (950,000) receiving antiretroviral therapy – bringing the total number of recipients to almost 3 million. The latter figure was the target of the '3 by 5' initiative that sought to have 3 million HIV-positive individuals living in low-and middle-income countries on treatment by 2005. Although that target was not achieved until two years later, it is widely credited with jump-starting the push towards ART scale-up.

According to the report, the rapid scale-up of ART can be attributed to a number of factors, including the:
⇨ Increased availability of drugs, in large part because of price reductions;
⇨ Improved ART delivery systems that are now better adapted to country contexts. The WHO public health approach to scale-up emphasises simplified and standardised drug regimens, decentralised services and judicious use of personnel and laboratory infrastructure; and
⇨ Increased demand for ART as the number of people who are tested and diagnosed with HIV climbs.

Greater access: greater need

The authors state that overall, some 31% of the estimated 9.7 million people in need of ART received it by the end of 2007. That means that an estimated 6.7 million in need are still unable to access life-saving medicines.

'This report highlights what can be achieved despite the many constraints that countries face and is a real step forward towards universal access to HIV prevention, treatment care and support,' said Dr Peter Piot, Executive Director of UNAIDS. 'Building on this, countries and the international community must now also work together to strengthen both prevention and treatment efforts.'

Preventing HIV in children

At the end of 2007, nearly 500,000 women were able to access anti-retrovirals to prevent transmission to their unborn children – up from 350,000 in 2006. During the same period, 200,000 children were receiving ART, compared

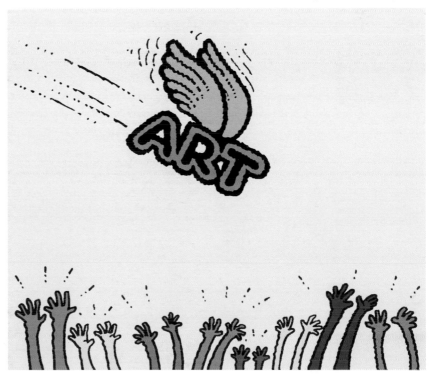

to 127,000 at the end of 2006. The difficulty of diagnosing HIV in infants, however, remains a major impediment to progress.

'We are seeing encouraging progress in the prevention of HIV transmission from mother to newborn,' said UNICEF Executive Director Ann M. Veneman. 'The report should motivate us to focus and redouble our efforts on behalf of children and families affected by HIV/AIDS.'

Tuberculosis, weak healthcare systems, hamper progress

Other obstacles to scaling up treatment include poor patient retention rates in many treatment programmes and the considerable numbers of individuals who remain unaware of their HIV status, or are diagnosed too late and die in the first six months of treatment.

Tuberculosis is a leading cause of death among HIV-infected people worldwide, and the number one cause of death among those living in Africa. To date, HIV and TB service deliveries are insufficiently integrated and too many people are losing their lives because they are unable to either prevent TB or access life-saving medications for both diseases.

The authors warn that future expansion of access to ART is likely to be slow owing to weak health systems in the worst-affected countries, in particular, the difficulty of training and retaining healthcare workers. Healthcare systems in regions hardest hit continue to erode because of 'brain drain' – the migration of skilled health-care personnel to other occupations and to other countries – and to high mortality rates from HIV itself.

They also emphasise the ongoing need to improve the collection, analysis and publication of critical public health information. Countries, international partners and other sources supply the numbers featured in this report. Despite certain limitations, the data constitute the best and most up-to-date estimates of the different elements of the health sector response to HIV/AIDS.
2 June 2008

⇨ The above information is reprinted with kind permission from the World Health Organisation. Visit www.who. int for more information.
© World Health Organisation

Fast facts about HIV treatment

Information from the World Health Organisation

In the early 1980s when the AIDS epidemic began, people living with HIV were not likely to live more than a few years. However, with the development of safe and effective drugs, HIV-positive people now have longer and healthier lives.

Currently available drugs do not cure HIV infection, but they do prevent the development of AIDS. They can stop the virus being made in the body and this stops the virus from damaging the immune system, but these drugs cannot eliminate HIV from the body. Hence, people with HIV need to continuously take antiretroviral drugs.

The use of antiretroviral (ARV) therapy in combinations of three or more drugs as an HIV treatment has dramatically improved the quality of life for people with HIV and prevented them from dying early, since 1996 in countries where they are widely accessible.

How does HIV treatment – or antiretroviral (ARV) therapy – work in someone who is HIV-positive?
HIV is a virus that infects cells of the human immune system and destroys or impairs their function. Infection with this virus results in the progressive deterioration of the immune system, leading to 'immune deficiency'. Our immune systems are essential to protect us from developing infections and cancers.

Combination ARV therapy prevents the HIV virus from multiplying inside a person. If this growth stops,

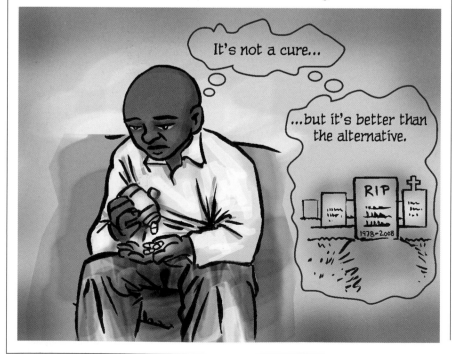

then the body's immune cells – most notably the CD4 cells – are able to live longer and provide the body protection from infections.

What is treatment adherence and why is it important?

HIV is a very active virus that makes lots of copies of itself that then damage the body's immune cells (CD4 cells). It is also a very clever virus that quickly adapts to whatever medicines are being taken as it tries to change itself through mutations so that these medicines no longer work.

However, taking at least 3 medicines at the same time makes it harder for the virus to adapt and become resistant. Taking the medicines every day at the right time and in the right way keeps the right levels of the medicines in the body, which makes it very hard for the virus to become resistant to the medicines. Missing your medication can give the HIV a chance to become resistant to the ARV medicine.

What are the side effects of HIV treatment?

Current World Health Organisation (WHO) recommendations for HIV treatment state that three separate ARV medicines need to be taken at all times.

Some of these medicines can produce side effects such as nausea and vomiting or headaches. Usually most side effects are not serious and improve once the patient gets used to the medicines. However, as with all medicines, sometimes unpleasant or dangerous side effects can appear. Some specific ARV medicines cause longer-term changes in body shape and the distribution of fat within the body, which can be upsetting for the patient. Usually changing the ARV medicines will lead to improvement in the patient's well-being.

How can ART prevent mother-to-child transmission of HIV?

HIV can pass from the mother to her unborn baby during pregnancy or the delivery and it can also be transferred to the baby by the mother's breast milk. This is usually called mother-to-child transmission of HIV (MTCT). Luckily we have a range of different things that can be done to prevent this, so it is important to make sure that all pregnant women have an HIV test.

If a pregnant woman does have HIV, first the doctors check to see if she needs treatment (ART) herself. If she does need ART then this is a very good way to make sure that her baby will not get the HIV. If she does not need ART herself, the mother will need to have ARV medicines during the pregnancy and the delivery to try to prevent the HIV from being passed to the baby.

Increasingly, people living with HIV are kept well and productive for very extended periods, even in low income countries

---

Once the baby is born, the mother needs to consider if replacement feeding – such as using mothers' milk substitutes – is a safe, feasible and acceptable long-term option for her and the family. If it is not, she needs to exclusively breastfeed the baby until replacement feeding becomes possible. All mothers need access to clear information, support and counselling when making these difficult choices.

The ARV regimens used to prevent transmission usually contain nevirapine or zidovudine (often known as AZT). Using only nevirapine may be the only option when women come very late to pregnancy care, but is not the best option to prevent transmission. In most high-income countries the rate of transmission of HIV to babies has been reduced to less than 1% by using a range of medicine and good care for the mother during pregnancy. HIV-positive women wanting to get pregnant are advised to do so in consultation with the health care provider to reduce the likelihood of their baby becoming infected.

Is there a cure for HIV?

No, there is no cure for HIV. However, with good and continued adherence to treatment the progression of the HIV in the body can be slowed down and almost halted. Increasingly, people living with HIV are kept well and productive for very extended periods, even in low-income countries.

What are antiretroviral drugs?

Antiretroviral drugs are used in the treatment and prevention of HIV infection. They work against HIV by stopping or interfering with the reproduction of virus in the body.

How do antiretroviral drugs work?

Inside an infected cell, HIV multiplies and produces lots of copies of itself, which can then go on to infect other healthy cells within the body. The more cells HIV infects, the greater is its impact on the immune system, and the more severe the deficiency in the immune system it produces (immunodeficiency). Antiretroviral drugs interfere with the way HIV makes copies of itself and the way it spreads from cell to cell. There are several different classes of drugs.

⇨ Nucleoside Reverse Transcriptase Inhibitors: HIV needs a substance called reverse transcriptase to make new copies of its genetic material (i.e. itself). This group of drugs inhibits this reverse transcriptase.

⇨ Non-Nucleoside Reverse Transcriptase Inhibitors: This group of drugs also blocks the reverse transcriptase.

⇨ Protease Inhibitors: HIV needs another substance called protease to be able to make new copies of itself. The protease inhibitors block this substance and so stop HIV multiplying.

Other drugs are also available that interfere with other steps in the process HIV uses to make copies of itself.

What is the difference between 'first', 'second' and 'third line' antiretroviral drugs?

HIV is a clever virus that quickly adapts to whatever medicines are being taken and tries to change itself through mutations so that these medicines no longer work and then the virus can start to reproduce to the same extent as before.

The first combination of drugs taken by a patient is usually called the first line regimen and when this no longer works to block HIV, another regimen made up of new medicines is needed. This is usually not needed for many years, and is called the second line regimen. If this also eventually fails, a third line or salvage cocktail of medicines is usually recommended.

What is the current status of ARV treatment?

Approximately three million people in low- and middle-income countries were receiving HIV antiretroviral therapy at the end of 2007.

Until 2003, the high cost of the medicines, weak or inadequate health care infrastructure and lack of financing prevented wide use of combination ART treatment in low- and middle-income countries.

However, enormous progress has been made and the increased political and economic commitment, stimulated by people living with HIV, civil society and other partners, has allowed dramatic expansion of access to HIV therapy.

What other kinds of care do people living with HIV need?

Even when ART is available, people living with HIV need other elements of care. In addition to access to HIV treatment, good nutrition, safe water, basic hygiene and other important elements of care can help maintain a high quality of life for a person living with HIV. Often people with HIV need psychosocial support and counselling.

Before ART is needed people usually are asked to start on cotrimoxazole or may need to take isoniazid to prevent TB.

What is 'PEP'?

The term 'post-exposure prophylaxis for HIV' (PEP) refers to a set of actions aimed at preventing infection in a person who may have been exposed to the HIV infection. It includes first aid care, counselling and risk assessment, HIV testing following informed consent, and – depending on the risk assessment – the provision of a short course (28 days) of antiretroviral drugs, with follow-up and support.

Research studies suggest that, if the medication is initiated quickly after possible HIV exposure, it may be beneficial in preventing HIV infection. However, PEP treatment has not been proven to prevent the transmission of HIV.

PEP should be available as soon as possible and no later than 72 hours, and be given for 28 days without interruption.

When you are on antiretroviral therapy, can you transmit the virus to others?

Taking antiretroviral therapy does not guarantee the prevention of transmission to sexual partners, infants or persons sharing unsafe injecting equipment. Usually ART keeps the HIV at very low levels or undetectable, but poor adherence, other illnesses, taking other medicines that interfere with levels of ARVs can mean the ART is not working well enough to prevent HIV being passed to others at risk.

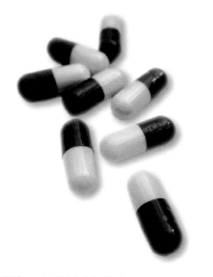

What is 'HAART'?

The term 'Highly Active Anti-Retroviral Therapy' (HAART) is another term used to describe a combination of three or more anti-HIV drugs.

Are the UNAIDS Secretariat and Cosponsors working with generic companies?

Yes they are. WHO and the UNAIDS Secretariat promote the engagement of both generic and research-based pharmaceutical companies in the response to HIV. WHO and UNAIDS co-hosted meetings in 2002 and

2003 and continue to work with drug firms.

A number of generic companies, in addition to research and development-based pharmaceuticals, have submitted applications and have been reviewed by the quality assessment project (known as 'pre-qualification') undertaken by WHO, with support from UNICEF and the UNAIDS Secretariat. Products from both branded and generic manufacturers that have met the international standards used by WHO in its 'prequalification' exercise are available at: http://www.who.int/prequal/query/ProductRegistry.aspx?list=ha

Generic drugs, diagnostics and other commodities have also been included in the published mapping of sources and prices of HIV-related medications undertaken by WHO, UNICEF, Médecins Sans Frontières and the UNAIDS Secretariat.

Representatives of the generic pharmaceutical industry, along with research-based companies, have participated in the Contact Group on Accelerating Access to AIDS-related care.

What is UNAIDS position regarding the exporting of generic drugs (including ARV medicines)?

UNAIDS supports the engagement of a broad range of partners in the response to the AIDS epidemic. Large volumes of antiretroviral medicines will be required to scale up access to treatment, and both research-based and generic manufacturers must be engaged.

The Declaration of Commitment unanimously endorsed by Member States at the UN 2001 General Assembly Special Session on HIV/AIDS emphasises the importance of cooperation in strengthening pharmaceutical policies and practices, including those applicable to generic drugs. The WHO Medicines Strategy includes promotion of generic competition.
June 2008

⇨ The above information is reprinted with kind permission from the World Health Organisation. Visit www.who.int for more information.
© World Health Organisation

Hope: an overlooked tool in the HIV/AIDS battle

Information from the Economic and Social Research Council

The links between HIV transmission and the degree to which people are able to adopt realistic plans to achieve future projects, in other words, hope, have been overlooked in policies to tackle HIV/AIDS. New research funded by the Economic and Social Research Council (ESRC) argues that hope is a powerful tool in the battle to stop the spread of HIV/AIDS.

Almost 30 years into the AIDS epidemic a medical vaccine for the disease remains elusive. Efforts to control the spread of HIV have been fairly successful in Western countries but have met little success in Africa. For example, life expectancy at birth is now estimated to be 36 years in Botswana, instead of 71 years without AIDS. It is expected to drop towards 30 within the next ten years.

ESRC Professorial Fellow, Tony Barnett, from the London School of Economics, argues: 'Current policies to tackle HIV/AIDS in Africa emphasise individual behaviour such as the ABC approach to prevention: Abstain, Be faithful, Condomise. However, these measures require that people have hope for the future and goals to aim for. And if wider economic and social circumstances are so poor that people lack hope for the future, then these current policies will have limited success.'

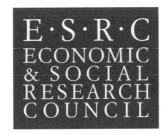

People with hope for the future are less likely to engage in activities in the present that put them at risk of illness in the future. Those without hope for the future, by contrast, place a low value on the future. For example, men who lack hope for the future may be unwilling to surrender immediate pleasure in return for a far-off future benefit by wearing a condom.

Increasing evidence shows that policies to combat AIDS that focus exclusively on individual behaviour are flawed if they dissociate behavioural change from the social, economic and cultural contexts. Security, stability, expectations of seeing the birth of grandchildren and their coming to adulthood, expectations of seeing a small enterprise grow bigger or a tree crop plantation come to maturity – these are all signs and indicators of hope that can have vital impacts on decisions and behaviours.

In contrast HIV/AIDS can destroy hope, resulting in vicious spirals that damage societies and lead to further HIV infections. When life prospects are so poor, people have little incentive to save for the future and to educate children. AIDS has also led to a growing number of orphans in Africa. Without financial, educational and emotional support for the future, a growing number of young people in Africa are less prepared for life and more vulnerable to HIV/AIDS.

'Hope is quite straightforward to measure via questionnaires and surveys can help to identify high risk environments,' concludes Professor Barnett. 'Although there is not a great deal of experience in developing programmes to increase hope, policies such as cash support for children, microfinance for small businesses, women's education, reduced discriminations against sexual minorities and health system reform will improve the wider environment. And with more to live for, interventions to encourage individuals to change their behaviour are more likely to succeed.'
8 August 2008

⇨ The above information is reprinted with kind permission from the Economic and Social Research Council. Visit www.esrcsocietytoday.ac.uk for more information.

© ESRC

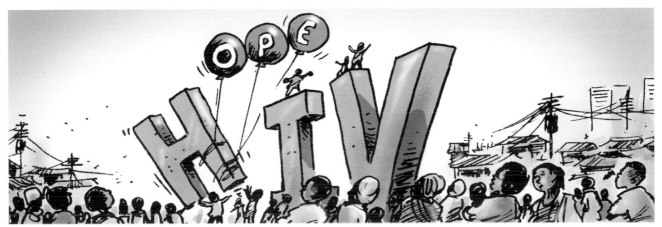

Is it time to give up the search for an AIDS vaccine?

After 25 years and billions of pounds, leading scientists are now forced to ask this question

Most scientists involved in AIDS research believe that a vaccine against HIV is further away than ever and some have admitted that effective immunisation against the virus may never be possible, according to an unprecedented poll conducted by *The Independent*.

A mood of deep pessimism has spread among the international community of AIDS scientists after the failure of a trial of a promising vaccine at the end of last year. It was just the latest in a series of setbacks in the 25-year struggle to develop an HIV vaccine.

The Independent's survey of more than 35 leading AIDS scientists in Britain and the United States found that just two were now more optimistic about the prospects for an HIV vaccine than they were a year ago; only four said they were more optimistic now than they were five years ago.

Nearly two-thirds believed that an HIV vaccine will not be developed within the next 10 years and some of them said that it may take at least 20 more years of research before a vaccine can be used to protect people either from infection or the onset of AIDS.

A substantial minority of the scientists admitted that an HIV vaccine may never be developed, and even those who believe that one could appear within the next 10 years added caveats saying that such a vaccine would be unlikely to work as a truly effective prophylactic against infection by the virus.

One of the major conclusions to emerge from the failed clinical trial of the most promising prototype vaccine, manufactured by the drug company Merck, was that an important animal model used for more than a decade, testing HIV vaccines on monkeys before they are used on humans, does not in fact work.

By Steve Connor and Chris Green

This has meant that prototype HIV vaccines which appear to work well when tested on monkeys infected with an artificial virus do not work when tested on human volunteers at risk of HIV – a finding that will be exploited by anti-vivisectionist campaigners opposed to vaccine experiments on primates.

> **Most scientists involved in AIDS research believe that a vaccine against HIV is further away than ever and some have admitted that effective immunisation against the virus may never be possible**

Anthony Fauci, the director of the US National Institute of Allergy and Infectious Diseases (NIAID), near Washington, told *The Independent*

that the animal model – which uses genetically engineered simian and human immunodeficiency viruses in a combination, known as SHIV – failed to predict what will happen when a prototype vaccine is moved from laboratory monkeys to people. 'We've learnt a few important things [from the clinical trial]. We've learnt that one of the animal models, the SHIV model, really doesn't predict very well at all,' he said.

'At least we now know that you can get a situation where it looks like you are protecting against SHIV and you're not protecting at all in the human model – that's important,' he said.

The NIAID spends about $500m (£250m) on HIV vaccine research each year and despite calls from some AIDS pressure groups for funds to be diverted to other forms of AIDS prevention, Dr Fauci said this was not the time to stop vaccine research. 'I don't think you should say that this is the point where we're going to give up on developing a vaccine. I think you continue given that there are so many unanswered questions to answer,' he said. 'There is an impression given by some that if you do vaccine research you are neglecting other areas of prevention. That's not

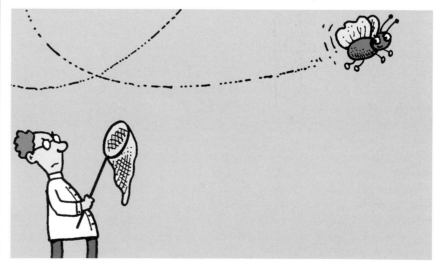

HIV diagnoses in young adults

UK HIV diagnoses in young adults (16-24) by year of diagnosis and exposure category: 1992 and earlier-2008

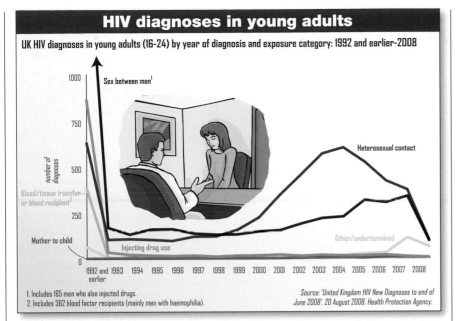

1. Includes 165 men who also injected drugs.
2. Includes 362 blood factor recipients (mainly men with haemophilia).

Source: 'United Kingdom HIV New Diagnoses to end of June 2008'. 20 August 2008. Health Protection Agency.

the case. We should and we are doing them simultaneously.'

More than 80 per cent of the scientists who took part in our survey agreed that it was now important to change the direction of HIV vaccine research, given the failure of the Merck clinical trial, which was cancelled when it emerged that the vaccine may have actually increased the chances of people developing AIDS.

Robert Gallo, a prominent AIDS researcher in the US who is credited with co-discovering the virus in the early 1980s, likened the vaccine's failure to the *Challenger* disaster, which forced Nasa to ground the space shuttle fleet for years.

At the end of last month, Dr Fauci convened a high-level summit of leading HIV specialists at a hotel in Bethesda, Maryland, to discuss the future direction of research. A group of 14 prominent AIDS specialists had already written to Dr Fauci suggesting that his institute had 'lost its way' in terms of an HIV vaccine.

He said that one outcome of the meeting was a refocusing of the vaccine effort away from expensive clinical trials towards more fundamental research to understand the basic biology of the virus and its effects on the human immune system.

'We'll be turning the knob more towards answering some fundamental questions rather than going into big clinical trials,' Dr Fauci said. 'I'm certainly disappointed that we're not further ahead in the development of a vaccine but I don't say that this year

I'm more discouraged than I was last year. I always knew from the beginning that it would be a very difficult task given what we know about this very elusive virus.'

About 33 million people in the world are infected with HIV and some 26 million have died of AIDS since the pandemic began.

The majority of scientists who responded to *The Independent*'s survey said that a vaccine would be the most effective way of preventing the spread of the virus given the failure of many education programmes.

Winnie Sseruma, 46: 'For me, the key has been not to give up'

Ms Sseruma says she believes abandoning research for a vaccine would mean a loss of hope for millions of people. 'When I was diagnosed, nearly 20 years ago, it was when the first drugs had come on the market. A lot of people had said before then that there was no hope and that all efforts should be put into prevention. But look where we are now. We cannot lose hope; we need to invest in a vaccine.'

She says this latest failure needs to be seen as the first hurdle, not a signal to give up. 'Yes, the scientists have not been very successful in their quest for a vaccine, but you can learn a lot from failures. Now they have realised they cannot use the normal routes used to develop simpler vaccines.'

Ms Sseruma lives in London, but was born in Uganda and says that the

current climate of pessimism for the vaccine is not dissimilar to the initial doubts over the likelihood of treating HIV in Africa.

'I remember when treatment started being available in the West and people were saying it would be impossible to send it to Africa. But look what's happened. We should always do whatever is humanly possible to fight AIDS. It's been a long journey, but for me, the key has been not to give up, and the scientists need to have the same attitude.'

'Philippe B', 42: 'People are getting resistant to drugs'

'Philippe', who wishes to remain anonymous, discovered he was HIV-positive 11 years ago. The 42-year-old believes the search for the vaccination should no longer be a priority, but that it should not stop altogether.

'Unfortunately what's happening now is that people are getting more resistant to drug treatment, and more money needs to be put into finding more drugs for treatment,' he said.

For people like Philippe, the fear of building an immunity to drugs and running out of options is a real one. He believes that as long as scientists are still pessimistic about the chances of successfully finding a vaccine, money needs to be invested in continuing to fund research into treatment.

'I've already become resistant to five combination treatments over the last ten years, and if I was on the last one available I'd be very afraid. HIV is not a death sentence in the way it once was, but we do need to fund further research into the drugs that treat it.'

Nevertheless, Philippe thinks it is not yet time to abandon all research into a vaccine. 'In my lifetime I don't think we'll have a vaccine, but there's no reason we should believe it isn't possible,' he said. 'But we should now be spending more on other ways of dealing with the disease.'
March 2008

⇨ The above information is reprinted with kind permission from Positive Nation. Visit www.positivenation.co.uk for more information.

© *Sugar media*

Inching closer

Despite setbacks, the search for an AIDS vaccine goes on. One day, we expect to be able to effectively protect people from this disease

By Seth Berkley

If you've been reading recent media coverage on AIDS vaccine research, such as the article in *The Independent* on 24 April, you might think developing an AIDS vaccine is a mission doomed to fail. If one setback always provoked that much pessimism about scientific efforts, developing new medicines and vaccines to address the world's ills would be an impossibly frustrating business. Fortunately, researchers are not so easily knocked off course. They know that breakthroughs are a product of patience and perseverance.

The latest media interest in AIDS vaccine research and development follows on recent discussions within the science community on how that work should continue in the wake of disappointing results in a clinical trial that tested a vaccine candidate made by Merck & Co. No serious scientists have suggested giving up on the effort to develop an AIDS vaccine. While it is impossible to predict with certainty a successful outcome, there is strong scientific evidence indicating that HIV can be controlled and infection prevented by activating the right immune response with the right vaccine.

Today, on the 10th World AIDS Vaccine Day, 25 years since the discovery of HIV, why do we not yet have an AIDS vaccine? I think many forget that AIDS vaccine work is a relatively young and pioneering science. Following disappointing results in the early 1980s, the effort withered. Serious investment and access to resources, including scientific expertise and research infrastructure in the countries most affected by AIDS, has only been available since the late 1990s.

What's more, scientists must explore new ways of designing vaccines for HIV because conventional methods are not appropriate. For instance, the 'live-attenuated' or 'whole-killed' virus approach, which uses a weakened or killed virus that cannot cause infection, is very effective in vaccines such as those against polio, measles and influenza. But this approach is not considered safe for HIV, out of concern that the crippled virus would not be adequately inactivated or could revert to its disease-causing form.

But that is not to say that AIDS vaccine researchers have not already made advances. We have learned a great deal about HIV – arguably more than about any other pathogen – and about its interaction with our immune system. Only in recent years have scientists from around the world begun to collaborate to turn this knowledge into novel designs for HIV vaccine candidates. Importantly, developing countries are playing a crucial role in this effort, following significant investment there in the infrastructure, scientists and technicians necessary to conduct clinical research.

With 33 million people living with HIV around the world, and 2.5 million newly infected last year, it is clear that existing interventions are not successfully controlling this pandemic, especially not in developing countries, which account for 95% of new infections. Investing in AIDS vaccine research is investing in an opportunity not just to ameliorate the suffering caused by AIDS but to actually end the epidemic. Certainly, that investment should not be at the expense of scaling up access to proven prevention strategies or of delivering much needed medication to people infected with HIV. Still, we cannot afford to neglect the vaccine effort. Vaccines remain the most powerful tool we have to control infectious diseases.

Almost certainly there is a long way to go before we will have an effective AIDS vaccine, but that is not news in vaccine development. It took decades for other vaccines, such as those against smallpox and polio, to be developed. Today, no one questions whether it was worth investing in these vaccines; most of us have been vaccinated and we live free from fear of infection by many deadly bacteria and viruses. Given the commitment of those who are in this field, I expect the same will be said one day of HIV.
18 May 2008

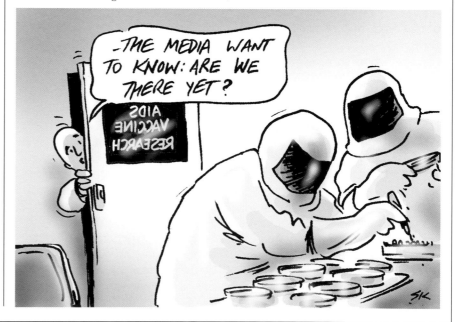

A cure for AIDS

Information from AVERT

There is no cure for AIDS. Although antiretroviral treatment can suppress HIV – the virus that causes AIDS – and can delay illness for many years, it cannot clear the virus completely. There is no confirmed case of a person getting rid of HIV infection. Sadly, this doesn't stop countless quacks and con artists touting unproven, often dangerous 'AIDS cures' to desperate people.

It is easy to see why an HIV-positive person might want to believe in an AIDS cure. Access to antiretroviral treatment is scarce in much of the world. When someone has a life-threatening illness they may clutch at anything to stay alive. And even when antiretroviral treatment is available, it is far from an easy solution. Drugs must be taken every day for the rest of a person's life, often causing unpleasant side effects. A one-off cure to eradicate the virus once and for all is much more appealing.

Distrust of Western medicine is not uncommon, especially in developing countries. The Internet abounds with rumours of the pharmaceutical industry or the US government suppressing AIDS cures to protect the market for patented drugs. Many people would prefer a remedy that is 'natural' or 'traditional'.

Where's the harm in fake AIDS cures?

Unproven AIDS cures have been around since the syndrome emerged in the early 1980s. In most cases, they have only served to worsen suffering.

First of all, fake cures are a swindle. Someone who invests their savings in a worthless potion or an electrical zapper has less money to spend on real medicines and healthy food.

Many peddlers of bogus cures insist their clients avoid all other treatments, including antiretroviral medicines. By the time a patient realises the 'cure' hasn't worked, their prospects for successful antiretroviral treatment may well have diminished.

Fake cures may also cause direct harm to health. Inventors often refuse to reveal their recipes. Some so-called cures have been found to contain industrial solvents, disinfectants and other poisons. The dangers posed by the virgin cleansing myth – which advocates sex with children as a cure for AIDS – are only too clear.

Finally, the promotion of fake AIDS cures undermines HIV prevention. People who believe in a cure are less likely to fear becoming infected with HIV, and hence less likely to take precautions.

Why is it so difficult to cure AIDS?

Curing AIDS is generally taken to mean clearing the body of HIV, the virus that causes AIDS. The virus replicates (makes new copies of itself) by inserting its genetic code into human cells, particularly a type known as CD4 cells. Usually the infected cells produce numerous HIV particles and die soon afterwards. Antiretroviral drugs interfere with this replication process, which is why the drugs are so effective at reducing the amount of HIV in a person's body to extremely low levels. During treatment, the concentration of HIV in the blood often falls so low that it cannot be detected by the standard test, known as a viral load test.

Unfortunately, not all infected cells behave the same way. Probably the most important problem is posed by 'resting' CD4 cells. Once infected with HIV, these cells, instead of producing new copies of the virus, lie dormant for many years or even decades. Current therapies cannot remove HIV's genetic material from these cells. Even if someone takes antiretroviral drugs for many years they will still have some HIV hiding in various parts of their body. Studies have found that if treatment is removed then HIV can re-establish itself by leaking out of these 'viral reservoirs'.

A cure for AIDS must somehow remove every single one of the infected cells.

Reputable research on curing AIDS

A wide range of strategies – including such drastic measures as bone marrow transplantation – have failed in trials to eradicate HIV infection. Currently, many researchers believe the best approach is to combine antiretroviral treatment with drugs that flush HIV from its hiding places. The idea is to force resting CD4 cells to become active, whereupon they will start producing new HIV particles. The activated cells should soon die or be destroyed by the immune system, and the antiretroviral medication should mop up the released HIV.

Early attempts to employ this technique used interleukin-2 (also known as IL-2 or by the brand name Proleukin). This chemical messenger tells the body to create more CD4 cells and to activate resting cells. Researchers who gave interleukin-2 together with antiretroviral treatment discovered they could no longer find any infected resting CD4 cells. But interleukin-2 failed to clear all of the HIV; as soon as the patients stopped taking antiretroviral drugs the virus came back again.

There is a problem with creating a massive number of active CD4 cells: despite the antiretroviral drugs, HIV may manage to infect a few of these cells and replicate, thus keeping the infection alive. Scientists are now investigating chemicals that don't activate all resting CD4 cells, but only the tiny minority that are infected with HIV.

One such chemical is valproic acid, a drug already used to treat epilepsy and other conditions. In 2005, a group of researchers led by David Margolis caused a sensation when they reported that valproic acid, combined with antiretroviral treatment, had greatly reduced the number of HIV-infected resting CD4 cells in three of four patients. They concluded that:

'This finding, though not definitive, suggests that new approaches will allow the cure of HIV in the future.'

Sadly, it seems such optimism was premature; more recent studies suggest that valproic acid has no long-term benefits. In fact it's quite possible that all related approaches are flawed because the virus has other hiding places besides resting CD4 cells. There is a lot about HIV that remains unknown.

Some of the world's top research institutions are today engaged in studies to learn more about the behaviour of HIV, resting CD4 cells and other hiding places. But the truth is that this field does not receive a lot of funding. Some people think the search for a cure is not worth much investment because the task may well be impossible.

Yet there are still those who remain hopeful, including the research charity amfAR, which in 2006 awarded nearly $1.5 million to AIDS cure researchers. Activist Martin Delaney is among those calling for an end to defeatism:

'Far too many people with HIV, as well as their doctors, have accepted the notion that a cure is not likely. No one can be certain that a cure will be found. No one can predict the future. But one thing is certain: if we allow pessimism about a cure to dominate our thinking, we surely won't get one... We must restore our belief in a cure and make it one of the central demands of our activism.'

⇨ The above information is reprinted with kind permission from AVERT. Visit www.avert.org for more.

© AVERT

Turning back the epidemic

New HIV infections and AIDS-related deaths declining – however, AIDS epidemic not over in any part of the world

According to new data in the UNAIDS 2008 *Report on the global AIDS epidemic* there have been significant gains in preventing new HIV infections in a number of heavily-affected countries. In Rwanda and Zimbabwe, changes in sexual behaviour have been followed by declines in the number of new HIV infections.

Condom use is increasing among young people with multiple partners in many countries. Another encouraging sign is that young people are waiting longer to have sexual intercourse. This has been seen in seven of the most affected countries: Burkina Faso, Cameroon, Ethiopia, Ghana, Malawi, Uganda and Zambia. In Cameroon the percentage of young people having sex before the age of 15 has gone down from 35% to 14%.

From 2005 to 2007 the percentage of HIV-positive pregnant women receiving antiretroviral drugs to prevent mother-to-child transmission (PMTCT) went up from 14% to 33%. In this same period the number of new infections among children fell from 410,000 to 370,000.

Several countries such as Argentina, the Bahamas, Barbados, Belarus, Cuba, Botswana, Georgia, Molodova, the Russian Federation and Thailand have achieved close to universal access with more than 75% coverage of PMTCT.

The report shows that the combined will and efforts of governments, donors, civil society and affected communities can make a difference.

Some 105 countries have set goals and targets towards achieving universal access to HIV prevention, treatment, care and support by 2010.

'Gains in saving lives by preventing new infections and providing treatment to people living with HIV must be sustained over the long term,' said UNAIDS Executive Director Dr Peter Piot. 'Short-term gains should serve as a platform for reinvigorating combination HIV prevention and treatment efforts and not spur complacency.'

The epidemic globally

From 2001 new HIV infections declined from 3 million to 2.7 million in 2007 [ranges: 2.6–3.5 million to 2.2–3.2 million]. Although the number of new HIV infections has fallen in several countries, the AIDS epidemic is not over in any part of the world.

Rates of new HIV infections are rising in many countries, such as China, Indonesia, Kenya, Mozambique, Papua New Guinea, the Russian Federation, Ukraine and Vietnam.

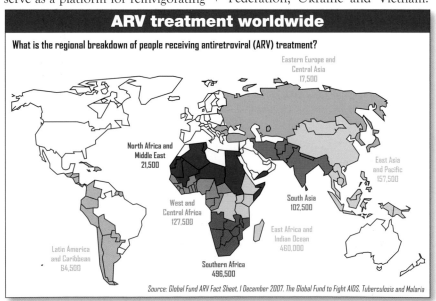

ARV treatment worldwide

What is the regional breakdown of people receiving antiretroviral (ARV) treatment?

Eastern Europe and Central Asia 17,500

North Africa and Middle East 21,500

East Asia and Pacific 157,500

West and Central Africa 127,500

South Asia 102,500

East Africa and Indian Ocean 460,000

Latin America and Caribbean 64,500

Southern Africa 496,500

Source: Global Fund ARV Fact Sheet, 1 December 2007. The Global Fund to Fight AIDS, Tuberculosis and Malaria

Increases in new HIV infections are also being seen in some older epidemics and HIV incidence is increasing in countries such as Germany, the United Kingdom and Australia.

⇨ An estimated 33.0 million [30.3–36.1 million] living with HIV worldwide.

⇨ 2.7 million [2.2 million–3.2 million] newly infected in 2007.

⇨ 2.0 million [1.8 million–2.3 million] died of AIDS in 2007.

The global epidemic has levelled off in terms of the percentage of people infected (prevalence), while the total number of people living with HIV has increased to 33 million people globally, with nearly 7,500 new infections each day.

Treatment is saving lives

As reported earlier in 2008, some 3 million people are now receiving antiretroviral treatment in low- and middle-income countries. Namibia scaled up treatment from 1% in 2003 to 88% in 2007. Similarly Cambodia scaled up treatment from 14% in 2004 to 67% in 2007. Other countries that have come close to achieving universal access to treatment are Botswana, Brazil, Chile, Costa Rica, Cuba and Lao People's Democratic Republic. In most parts of the world more women are receiving antiretroviral treatment than men.

In part as a result of the scaling up in the past two years, AIDS-related deaths have declined from 2.2 million to 2 million in 2007 [ranges: 1.9–2.6 million to 1.8–2.3 million].

However, AIDS continues to be the leading cause of death in Africa, which is home to 67% of all people living with HIV. In Africa, 60% of people living with HIV in the region are women and three out of four young people living with HIV are female.

More attention for people most at risk

Since 2005 there has been a tripling of HIV prevention efforts focused on sex workers, men who have sex with men and injecting drug users. For example, of the 39 countries reporting on access to HIV-prevention services for sex workers, there was a 60% average coverage rate. Nearly 50% of people who inject drugs in 15 countries and 40% of men who have sex with men in 27 countries had access to HIV-prevention services.

In virtually all regions outside of sub-Saharan Africa, HIV infections have disproportionately affected injecting drug users, men who have sex with men, and sex workers. People most at risk have better access to HIV prevention services in countries that have laws to protect them against discrimination.

'Knowing your local epidemic' remains critical to effective prevention efforts. Over time, trends have changed within regions and within countries. In Thailand the main mode of transmission was sex work and injecting drug use and now the main mode of transmission is among married couples.

'Countries need to focus HIV prevention programmes to where the new infections are occurring,' said UNFPA Executive Director Dr Thoraya Obaid. 'Knowing the epidemic and choosing the right combination of interventions are critical for an effective response. In many contexts, young people and women need special attention.'

Looking ahead

The new report is being launched ahead of the XVII International AIDS Conference in Mexico. This event will bring together leaders, policymakers, academics, activists, community groups and other key stakeholders to review lessons learnt and build momentum towards achieving universal access goals by 2010 and the Millennium Development Goals by 2015.

'Responding to AIDS is an important Millennium Development Goal which also has a direct impact on meeting the other Goals by 2015,' said UNDP Administrator Kemal Dervis. 'The progress we make in addressing AIDS will contribute to our efforts to reducing poverty and child mortality, and to improving nutrition and maternal health. At the same time, progress towards the other Goals, such as tackling gender inequality and promoting education, is required if we are to halt and reverse the spread of AIDS.'

Long-term response

AIDS is a long-term issue and one that requires a response that is grounded in evidence and human rights. It requires strong leadership that can sustain commitments over time. The report calls for leaders to approach issues of human sexuality and drug use with a human rights perspective.

HIV responses require long-term sustained financing. As more people go on treatment and live longer, budgets for HIV will have to increase over the next few decades. Donors will have to provide the majority of the funding required for the AIDS responses in low- and some middle-income countries, even as domestic spending on HIV has increased in these countries. The response will be helped by commitments such as the recent reauthorisation of US$ 48 billion by the United States Government. The G8, at its recent summit in Japan, also agreed to honour in full its commitments to continue working towards the goal of universal access to HIV prevention and treatment by 2010.

'The scaling up of the AIDS response towards universal access must be based on four key values – a rights-based approach, multisectoralism, results for people, and community engagement. These are not negotiable,' said Dr Piot.

About the UNAIDS 2008 report on the global AIDS epidemic

The 2008 *Report on the global AIDS epidemic*, prepared by UNAIDS and its cosponsoring agencies, is the most comprehensive report on the response to AIDS. It uses data from 147 countries against 25 core targets set in the UN declaration of commitment on HIV/AIDS adopted in 2001, and the political declaration adopted at the 2006 High Level Meeting on AIDS. The information presented in the report enables readers to assess progress made since 2001 and identify the strengths and weaknesses of the AIDS response to date.
29 July 2008

⇨ The above information is reprinted with kind permission from UNAIDS. Visit www.unaids.org for more information.

© *UNAIDS*

⇨ Worldwide figures estimate that over 40 million people are living with HIV and around three million people die each year from AIDS-related illnesses. (page 1)

⇨ There is no cure for HIV infection, but treatment with anti-HIV medicines dramatically slows the progress of the disease and has significantly reduced the number of deaths caused by AIDS-related illnesses. (page 2)

⇨ According to the latest (2008) WHO and UNAIDS global estimates, women comprise 50% of people living with HIV. (page 5)

⇨ Worldwide, over 15 million children under the age of 18 have lost one or both parents to AIDS – a number that is expected to reach 20 million by 2010. (page 6)

⇨ HIV-infected patients in high income countries are living some 13 years longer thanks to improvements in combination antiretroviral therapy (cART), according to new research. (page 8)

⇨ More people have been infected with HIV/AIDS by heterosexual sex than by any other method of transmission. (page 11)

⇨ The latest figures from the Health Protection Agency reveal that the number of people living with HIV in the UK increased to an estimated 77,400 in 2007, with 7,734 new diagnoses in 2007 alone. (page 16)

⇨ Heterosexually-acquired HIV infections, most of which were in immigrants and migrants, formed the largest proportion (42%) of new HIV infections diagnosed in Western Europe in 2006. A little under one-third (29%) of newly diagnosed HIV infections were attributable to unsafe sex between men, while a diminishing proportion of diagnoses (6%) were reported in injecting drug users. (page 17)

⇨ New research indicates that one in seven young people interviewed in Britain would not be willing to remain friends with someone if they had HIV and only 32% are worried about getting HIV. (page 18)

⇨ An estimated 73,000 adults are now living with HIV in the UK, according to the Health Protection Agency's latest report on the UK's sexual health. This figure includes both those who have been diagnosed and also around a third (21,600) who remain unaware of their HIV status. (page 22)

⇨ In 2007, over 90 per cent of the British public did not fully understand the ways that HIV is transmitted, with Scotland and London reportedly being the least knowledgeable regions. (page 23)

⇨ Only 1.2% of all HIV-positive women who gave birth in the UK between 2000 and 2006 passed their HIV infection to their child. (page 25)

⇨ Forty-nine per cent of the British public don't always use a condom when with a new sexual partner, according to the Ipsos MORI survey conducted for the National AIDS Trust (NAT). (page 26)

⇨ HIV can only be transmitted in a few ways: through sex, blood and mother-to-child transmission. (page 26)

⇨ Nearly three million people are now receiving antiretroviral therapy (ART) in low- and middle-income countries, according to a new report. (page 29)

⇨ The use of antiretroviral (ARV) therapy in combinations of three or more drugs as an HIV treatment has dramatically improved the quality of life for people with HIV and prevented them from dying early, since 1996 in countries where they are widely accessible. (page 30)

⇨ Efforts to control the spread of HIV have been fairly successful in Western countries but have met little success in Africa. For example, life expectancy at birth is now estimated to be 36 years in Botswana, instead of 71 years without AIDS. It is expected to drop towards 30 within the next ten years. (page 33)

⇨ Most scientists involved in AIDS research believe that a vaccine against HIV is further away than ever and some have admitted that effective immunisation against the virus may never be possible, according to an unprecedented poll conducted by The Independent. (page 34)

⇨ Developing countries account for 95% of new HIV infections. (page 36)

⇨ From 2005 to 2007 the percentage of HIV-positive pregnant women receiving antiretroviral drugs to prevent mother-to-child transmission (PMTCT) went up from 14% to 33%. In this same period the number of new infections among children fell from 410,000 to 370,000. (page 38)

⇨ AIDS continues to be the leading cause of death in Africa, which is home to 67% of all people living with HIV. In Africa, 60% of people living with HIV in the region are women and three out of four young people living with HIV are female. (page 39)

ABC strategy

This refers to a sex education policy developed in response to the HIV and AIDS epidemic in Africa – **A**bstinence, **B**e faithful, use a **C**ondom.

AIDS

Acquired Immune Deficiency Syndrome (AIDS) is diagnosed when the immune system has been weakened so much by HIV that it can't fight certain life-threatening infections and illnesses. It is fatal and cannot be cured.

Anti-retroviral therapy (ART)

While there is no cure for the HIV virus, ART medicines are very effective in controlling the illness, and can extend life expectancy considerably for those living with the disease. Unfortunately, ART treatments are not yet universally available, and are particularly hard to obtain in the developing world.

Criminal transmission

Transmission of HIV can be classed as intentional, reckless or accidental. Some people who have deliberately infected others with the virus (for example, by having unprotected sex with a partner who wrongly believes them to be HIV-negative) have been prosecuted in the courts.

Epidemics and pandemics

The prevalence and growth of the HIV virus may be referred to either as an epidemic or a pandemic. An epidemic refers to the number of new cases of a disease which appear within a given human population, when they are substantially beyond what might be expected. A pandemic refers to an epidemic of an infectious disease that spreads through populations across a large area, such as a continent.

HIV

Human Immunodeficiency Virus (HIV) is an infection. It can be passed from person to person via unprotected sex, from needles contaminated with infected blood, through blood transfusion or organ donation from people with the virus, and from mother to baby. HIV affects the body's immune system, weakening its ability to fight infection. It can be controlled through the use of anti-retroviral medicines, but there is no cure. Individuals living with the disease are referred to as HIV-positive.

IDU

Injecting drug users. These are an at-risk group for HIV transmission, as needles contaminated with infected blood may be shared between users. It is estimated that 131 injecting drug users became infected with HIV in the UK during 2006 – a fairly low number compared with some other countries.

Immune system

The immune system protects your body against infection. A key part is white blood cells. These cells find and destroy invading germs, such as bacteria and viruses, preventing the development of serious diseases and damage to your body. HIV avoids being destroyed by the immune system by repeatedly changing its outer 'coat'. It multiplies (replicates) within the special type of white blood cells called CD4 cells. These cells are normally involved in helping other types of immune cell to attack and destroy disease-causing germs. As HIV multiplies, it destroys CD4 cells, so there are less of them. The reduction in CD4 cells means that the body's ability to fight infection is weakened.

PMTCT

Preventing mother-to-child transmission. HIV can be passed from an HIV-positive mother to her baby during birth, and also via breast milk. However, if the mother is diagnosed as HIV-positive before giving birth, measures can be taken to ensure the risk of her transmitting HIV to her baby is very low. Only 1.2% of all HIV-positive women who gave birth in the UK between 2000 and 2006 passed their infection to their child.

MSM

Men who have sex with men. Since the beginning of the UK AIDS epidemic, men who have sex with men have been the group most at risk of HIV infection.

STI

STI stands for sexually-transmitted infection. HIV is classed as an STI.

INDEX

Additional Resources

Other Issues titles

If you are interested in researching further some of the issues raised in *The AIDS Crisis*, you may like to read the following titles in the **Issues** series:

⇨ Vol. 163 *Drugs in the UK* (ISBN 978 1 86168 456 1)

⇨ Vol. 153 *Sexual Orientation and Society* (ISBN 978 1 86168 440 0)

⇨ Vol. 152 *Euthanasia and the Right to Die* (ISBN 978 1 86168 439 4)

⇨ Vol. 123 *Young People and Health* (ISBN 978 1 86168 362 5)

⇨ Vol. 96 *Preventing Sexual Diseases* (ISBN 978 1 86168 304 5)

⇨ Vol. 81 *Alternative Therapies* (ISBN 978 1 86168 276 5)

For more information about these titles, visit our website at www.independence.co.uk/publicationslist

Useful organisations

You may find the websites of the following organisations useful for further research:

⇨ **ActionAid International:** www.actionaid.org.uk

⇨ **AVERT:** www.avert.org

⇨ **Global AIDS Alliance:** www.globalaidsalliance.org

⇨ **Health Protection Agency:** www.hpa.org.uk

⇨ **National AIDS Trust:** www.worldaidsday.org.uk

⇨ **Pfizer:** www.abouthivaids.org

⇨ **Positive Nation:** www.positivenation.co.uk

⇨ **Staying Alive:** www.staying-alive.org

⇨ **Terrence Higgins Trust:** www.tht.org.uk

⇨ **UNAIDS:** www.unaids.org

⇨ **World Health Organisation:** www.who.int

ACKNOWLEDGEMENTS

The publisher is grateful for permission to reproduce the following material.

While every care has been taken to trace and acknowledge copyright, the publisher tenders its apology for any accidental infringement or where copyright has proved untraceable. The publisher would be pleased to come to a suitable arrangement in any such case with the rightful owner.

Chapter One: The AIDS Epidemic

HIV / AIDS, © Bupa, *HIV / AIDS estimates are revised downwards*, © World Health Organisation, *Gender inequalities and HIV*, © World Health Organisation, *Protect the children*, © Global AIDS Alliance, *Life expectancy of HIV patients increases*, © University of Bristol, *Gay men with HIV have near-normal death rates*, © Sugar media, *HIV in developing countries*, © ActionAid International, *What do you know about HIV / AIDS?*, © Pfizer, *Criminal transmission of HIV*, © AVERT, *Diseased theories*, © Guardian Newspapers Limited.

Chapter Two: HIV/AIDS in the UK

Record UK HIV diagnoses, © National AIDS Trust, *AIDS epidemic update*, © WHO/UNAIDS, *Stigmatising HIV and AIDS*, © British Red Cross, *Step into the future*, Sugar media, *Getting tested for HIV*, © Staying Alive, *Living with HIV*, © Terrence Higgins Trust, *HIV and gay men*, © Health Protection Agency.

Chapter Three: Fighting HIV and AIDS

HIV prevention in the UK, © AVERT, *Condom use*, © Crown copyright is reproduced with the permission of Her Majesty's Stationery Office, *Stop HIV: beyond ABC*, © Global AIDS Alliance, *3 million now receiving life-saving HIV drugs*, © World Health Organisation, *Fast facts about HIV treatment*, © World Health Organisation, *Hope: an overlooked tool in the HIV/AIDS battle*, © Economic and Social Research Council, *Is it time to give up the search for an AIDS vaccine?*, © Sugar media, *Inching closer*, © Guardian Newspapers Limited, *A cure for AIDS*, © AVERT, *Turning back the epidemic*, © UNAIDS.

Photographs

Flickr: pages 16 (Jeremy Foo); 20 (Antonio).
Stock Xchng: pages 6 (Silvia Cosimini); 14 (Jason Morrison); 17 (Kym McLeod); 24 (Irineu I Degasperi); 32 (dima v).
Wikimedia Commons: pages 9 (Till Krech); 28 (ChristianHeldt).

Illustrations

Pages 3, 21, 29, 34: Don Hatcher; pages 11, 22, 30: Angelo Madrid; pages 12, 25, 33, 36: Simon Kneebone; pages 16, 26: Bev Aisbett.

Additional editorial by Claire Owen, on behalf of Independence Educational Publishers.

And with thanks to the team: Mary Chapman, Sandra Dennis, Claire Owen and Jan Sunderland.

Lisa Firth
Cambridge
January, 2009